METHODS AND TECHNIQUES FOR FIRE DETECTION

METHODS AND TECHNIQUES FOR FIRE DETECTION

Signal, Image and Video Processing Perspectives

A. ENIS ÇETIN

BART MERCI

OSMAN GÜNAY

BEHÇET UĞUR TÖREYİN

STEVEN VERSTOCKT

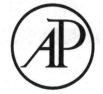

AMSTERDAM • BOSTON • HEIDELBERG • LONDON
NEW YORK • OXFORD • PARIS • SAN DIEGO
SAN FRANCISCO • SINGAPORE • SYDNEY • TOKYO
Academic Press is an imprint of Elsevier

Academic Press is an imprint of Elsevier
125 London Wall, London, EC2Y 5AS, UK
525 B Street, Suite 1800, San Diego, CA 92101-4495, USA
50 Hampshire Street, 5th Floor, Cambridge, MA 02139, USA
The Boulevard, Langford Lane, Kidlington, Oxford OX5 1GB, UK

Notices
Knowledge and best practice in this field are constantly changing. As new research and experience broaden our understanding, changes in research methods, professional practices, or medical treatment may become necessary.

Practitioners and researchers must always rely on their own experience and knowledge in evaluating and using any information, methods, compounds, or experiments described herein. In using such information or methods they should be mindful of their own safety and the safety of others, including parties for whom they have a professional responsibility.

To the fullest extent of the law, neither the Publisher nor the authors, contributors, or editors, assume any liability for any injury and/or damage to persons or property as a matter of products liability, negligence or otherwise, or from any use or operation of any methods, products, instructions, or ideas contained in the material herein.

Library of Congress Cataloging-in-Publication Data
A catalog record for this book is available from the Library of Congress

British Library Cataloguing-in-Publication Data
A catalogue record for this book is available from the British Library

ISBN: 978-0-12-802399-0

For information on all Academic Press publications
visit our website at http://store.elsevier.com/

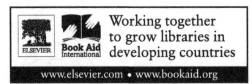

Working together
to grow libraries in
developing countries

www.elsevier.com • www.bookaid.org

Publisher: Joe Hayton
Acquisition Editor: Tim Pitts
Editorial Project Manager: Charlotte Kent
Production Project Manager: Jason Mitchell
Designer: Maria Inês Cruz

CONTENTS

BIOGRAPHY

A. Enis Çetin got his PhD degree from the University of Pennsylvania in 1987. Between 1987 and 1989, he was an assistant professor of electrical engineering at the University of Toronto. He has been with Bilkent University, Ankara, Turkey, since 1989. Çetin was an associate editor of IEEE Transactions on Image Processing between 1999 and 2003. Currently, he is on the editorial boards of IEEE Signal Processing Magazine, IEEE Transactions on Circuits and Systems for Video Technology, and Machine Vision and Applications (IAPR), Springer. He is the editor-in-chief of Signal, Image, and Video Processing, Springer. He is a fellow of IEEE. His research interests include signal and image processing, human–computer interaction using vision and speech, and audiovisual multimedia databases.

Bart Merci is full professor at Ghent University (Belgium). He is head of the research unit "Combustion, Fire and Fire Safety." Having completed a PhD (Ghent University, 2000) on turbulence modeling in CFD simulations of non-premixed combustion, he is an expert in fluid mechanics aspects in reacting flows, more particularly related to fire and smoke dynamics. He has already coauthored over 100 peer review publications and over 200 conference publications and is an editorial board member of multiple leading journals in the field. He initiated and coordinates the International Master of Science in Fire Safety Engineering, a collaboration of Ghent University, Lund University, and the University of Edinburgh, with the University of Queensland, ETH Zürich and University of Maryland as Associated Partners.

Osman Günay received his BSc and MS degrees in Electrical and Electronics Engineering from Bilkent University, Ankara, Turkey. In 2015, he received his PhD degree from the same department. Since 2011, he has been working in the defense industry as a system engineer. His research interests include computer vision, video segmentation, and dynamic texture recognition.

Behçet Uğur Töreyin received his BS degree from the Middle East Technical University, Ankara, Turkey, in 2001 and MS and PhD degrees from Bilkent University, Ankara, in 2003 and 2009, respectively, all in electrical and electronics engineering. He is now an Assistant Professor with the Informatics Institute at Istanbul Technical University. His research interests lie broadly in signal processing and pattern recognition with applications to image/video analysis, and communication systems. His research is focused on developing novel algorithms to analyze and compress signals from a multitude of sensors such as visible/infra-red/hyperspectral cameras, microphones, passive infra-red sensors, vibration sensors, and spectrum sensors for wireless communications.

Steven Verstockt received his master's degree in informatics from Ghent University in 2003. Following his studies in applied informatics, he began teaching Multimedia courses at Hogeschool Gent and at the end of 2007, he joined the ELIT Lab of the University College West-Flanders as a researcher. In 2008, he started a PhD on video fire analysis at the Multimedia Lab of the Department of Electronics and Information Systems of Ghent University—iMinds (Belgium). Since 2012, he has worked as a postdoctoral researcher in this lab focusing on multi-sensor fire analysis. In October 2015, he was appointed a tenure track position as assistant professor in Multimedia at the same lab.

ACKNOWLEDGMENTS

Research activities in this book were funded by the Turkish Scientific and Technical Research Council (TÜBİTAK), the European Commission 7th Framework Program under Grant FP7-ENV-2009-1244088 FIRESENSE (Fire Detection and Management through a Multi-Sensor Network for the Protection of Cultural Heritage Areas from the Risk of Fire and Extreme Weather Conditions), Ghent University, iMinds, the Institute for the Promotion of Innovation by Science and Technology in Flanders (IWT), the Fund for Scientific Research-Flanders, and the Belgian Federal Science Policy Office. A. Enis Çetin, Behçet Uğur Töreyin and Osman Günay would like to express their gratitude to Mr. Nurettin Doğan and Mr. İlhami Aydin of the Turkish General Directorate of Forestry (Orman Genel Müdürlüğü— OGM), and to Dr. M. Bilgay Akhan suggesting them to study computer vision based fire detection.

CHAPTER 1

Introduction

Signal, image, and video processing are widely used in many security applications. It is possible to use visible-range and special purpose infrared surveillance cameras as well as pyro-infrared detectors for fire detection. This requires intelligent signal processing techniques for detection and analysis of uncontrolled fire behavior. As the number of recently proposed signal, image, and video processing-based fire detection methods increased over the last 10 years, a need for a book presenting basic principles of these methods emerged.

This book describes signal, image, and video processing methods and techniques for fire detection. The intended audience of the book is graduate students, researchers, and practitioners working on signal processing and computer vision-based techniques for fire detection. The book provides them with a thorough and practical overview of the state-of-the-art methods and techniques in this domain.

Sensors enhanced with intelligent signal and image processing capabilities may help reduce the detection time compared to the currently available sensors for both indoors and outdoors. This is due to the fact that cameras and other nonconventional fire sensors can monitor "volumes" and do not have the transport delay that the traditional "point" sensors suffer from. For example, it is possible to cover an area of 100 km^2 using a single pan-tilt-zoom camera placed on a hilltop for wildfire detection. Another benefit of volumetric sensor systems is that they can provide crucial information about the size and growth of the fire and the direction of smoke propagation.

During the last decades, improvements in the computational power of computers and the decreasing cost of imaging sensors made it possible to employ video-based fire detection techniques for real-time applications. In the literature, video fire detection algorithms developed for visible range cameras are higher in number as visible range cameras cost less compared to infrared (thermal) and time-of-flight cameras. In Chapter 2, state-of-the-art camera-based techniques for fire detection are presented.

Chapter 3 presents a set of methods for flame detection using a nonconventional sensor, a pyro–electric infrared (PIR) sensor, which is a low-cost sensor widely used for motion detection. The methods are based on the

Methods and Techniques for Fire Detection
http://dx.doi.org/10.1016/B978-0-12-802399-0.00001-6

analysis of the flame flicker existing inherently in uncontrolled fires. The PIR sensors are commonly used for occupancy detection purposes in buildings. Utilizing techniques and methods presented in Chapter 3, they may turn into uncontrolled fire detectors as well.

Current methods and techniques used for multi-sensor fire analysis are described in Chapter 4. Methods in Chapter 4 are aimed at estimating the origin and growth of fires, rather than detecting them. Modeling fire behavior has important benefits in firefighting and mitigation, and is essential in assessing the risk of escalation. Techniques in Chapter 4 focus on multi-modal/multi-sensor analysis of fire characteristics, such as flame and smoke spread.

Surveillance cameras and PIR-based motion sensors are widely used in modern buildings. It is now possible to use them for fire and smoke detection by analyzing the video and signals that they generate. It is our hope that the methods and techniques discussed in this book will lead to safer buildings and living environments in the near future.

CHAPTER 2

Camera-Based Techniques

Contents

Part 1

The first step in video fire detection (VFD) is to apply a background subtraction algorithm to extract moving regions in the video. Then the detected regions are analyzed temporally to be classified in terms of flickering characteristics. Markov models and frequency domain techniques can be used to identify if the flickering characteristics belong to flames. In the next step, spatial analysis is performed to check for the irregularities that are used to identify flames.

Another method is to extract features from the moving regions and use classifiers who are trained offline with videos of fire and false alarm sources. It is also possible to use active learning algorithms which are updated online to classify flame regions. The most important problem with visible range fire detections is the false alarms. Fire-colored moving regions can be difficult to distinguish from the actual flames. Fire detection algorithms are generally developed for stationary cameras. When moving cameras are used, it becomes difficult to detect the flickering characteristics of flames. Detection of fire using a moving camera is a future research problem. Another application of video-based fire detection is smoke detection for early wildfire warning systems. Forests are usually monitored using PTZ cameras that scan recorded preset positions in a specific order. These cameras can monitor larger distances than usual visible range cameras. In wildfire detection applications, smoke becomes visible before the flames; therefore it makes sense to focus on smoke detection for these systems.

With the decreased cost of infrared sensors, it became possible to use long- and short-wave infrared cameras for flame detection. Since infrared (thermal) cameras form images whose intensity depend on the temperature of the objects, they could be used to reduce most of the false alarms. In most cases, the temperature of flames is higher than the surrounding environment and IR cameras can successfully detect the flickering flames. Initially, infrared flame detection algorithms processed near infrared images (NIR) to verify the existence of flames. More recent methods started to use short- and long-wave infrared (SWIR, LWIR) thermal cameras for fire and flame detection.

This chapter is based on the VFD survey paper in [1]. Recently proposed VFD techniques are viable alternatives or complements to existing fire detection techniques and have shown to be useful in solving several problems related to the traditional sensors. Conventional sensors are generally limited to indoors and are not applicable in large open spaces such as shopping centers, airports, car parks, and forests. They require a close proximity to the fire and most of them cannot provide additional information about fire location, dimension, etc. One of the main limitations of commercially available fire alarm systems is that it may take a long time for carbon particles and smoke to reach the "point" detector. This is called the "transport delay." It is our belief that video analysis can be applied in conditions in which conventional methods fail. VFD has the potential to detect the fire from a distance in large open spaces because cameras can monitor "volumes." As a result, VFD does not have the transport and threshold delay from which the traditional "point" sensors suffer. As soon as smoke or flames occur in one of the camera views, it is possible to detect fire immediately. We all know that human beings can detect an uncontrolled fire using their eyes and vision systems, but as pointed out above, it is not easy to replicate human intelligence.

The research in this domain was started in the late nineties. Most of the VFD articles available in the literature are influenced by the notion of "weak" Artificial Intelligence (AI) framework which was first introduced by Hubert L. Dreyfus in his critique of the "generalized" AI [3,4]. Dreyfus presents solid philosophical and scientific arguments on why the search for "generalized" AI is futile [5]. Therefore, each specific problem including VFD fire should be addressed as an individual engineering problem which has its own characteristics [6]. It is possible to approximately model the fire behavior in video using various signal and image processing methods and automatically detect fire based on the information extracted from video. However, the current systems suffer from false alarms because of modeling and training inaccuracies.

Currently available VFD algorithms mainly focus on the detection and analysis of smoke and flames in consecutive video images. In early articles, mainly flame detection was investigated. Recently, the smoke detection problem is also considered. The reason for this can be found in the fact that smoke spreads faster and in most cases will occur much faster in the field of view of the cameras. In wildfire applications, it may not even be possible to observe flames for a long time. The majority of the state-of-the-art detection techniques focuses on the color and shape characteristics, together with the temporal behavior of smoke and flames. However, due to the variability of shape, motion, transparency, colors, and patterns of smoke and flames, many of the existing VFD approaches are still vulnerable to false alarms. Due to noise, shadows, illumination changes, and other visual artifacts in recorded video sequences, developing a reliable detection system is a challenge to the image processing and computer vision community.

With today's technology, it is not possible to have a fully reliable VFD system without a human operator. However, current systems are invaluable tools for surveillance operators. It is also our strong belief that combining multi-modal video information using both visible and infrared (IR) technology will lead to higher detection accuracy. Each sensor type has its own specific limitations, which can be compensated by other types of sensors. Although, it would be desirable to develop a fire detection system which could operate on the existing closed circuit television (CCTV) equipment without introducing any additional cost. However, the cost of using multiple video sensors does not outweigh the benefit of multi-modal fire analysis. The fact that IR manufacturers also ensure a decrease in the sensor cost in the near future fully opens the door to multi-modal video analysis. VFD cameras can also be used to extract useful related information, such as the presence of people caught in the fire, fire size, fire growth, smoke direction, etc.

VFD systems can be classified into various subcategories according to
(i) the spectral range of the camera used,
(ii) the purpose (flame or smoke detection),
(iii) the range of the system.
There are overlaps between the categories above.

2.1 VFD IN VISIBLE/VISUAL SPECTRAL RANGE

Over the last years, the number of papers about visual fire detection in the computer vision literature has grown exponentially [2]. As is, this relatively new subject in vision research is in full progress and has already produced promising results. However, this is not a completely solved problem, as with most computer vision problems. Behavior of smoke and flames of an uncontrolled fire differs with distance and illumination. Furthermore, cameras are not color and/or spectral measurement devices. They have different sensors and color and illumination balancing algorithms. They may produce different images and video for the same scene because of their internal settings and algorithms.

In this section, a chronological overview of the state-of-the-art (ie, a collection of frequently referenced papers on short range [<100 m]) fire detection methods is presented in the tables below. For each of these papers, we investigated the underlying algorithms and checked the appropriate techniques. In the following, we discuss each of these detection techniques and analyze their use in the listed papers.

State-of-the-art: underlying techniques (PART1: 2002–2007).

Paper	Color detection	Moving object detection	Flicker/energy (wavelet) analysis	Spatial difference analysis	Dynamic texture/Pattern analysis	Disorder analysis	Subblocking	Training (models, NN, SVM, ...)	Cleanup post-processing	Localization/analysis	Flame detection	Smoke detection
Phillips [7]	RGB		X	X				X	X		X	
Gomez–Rodriguez [8]		X	X			X						X
Gomez–Rodriguez [9]		X	X			X						X
Chen [10]	RGB/HSI	X				X					X	X
Liu [11]	HSV		X			X					X	
Marbach [12]	YUV		X			X					X	
Toreyin [13]	RGB	X	X	X							X	X
Toreyin [14]	YUV	X	X			X						X
Celik [15]	YCbCr/RGB										X	
Xu [16]		X	X			X					X	X

State-of-the-art: underlying techniques (PART 2: 2007–2009).

Paper	Color detection	Moving object detection	Flicker/ energy (wavelet) analysis	Spatial difference analysis	Dynamic texture/ pattern analysis	Disorder analysis	Subblocking	Training (models, NN, SVM, ...)	Cleanup post-processing	Localization/ analysis	Flame detection	Smoke detection
Celik [17]	RGB	X				X		X	X		X	
Xiong [18]		X	X			X						X
Lee [19]	RGB	X	X					X	X		X	X
Calderara [20]	RGB	X	X				X	X				X
Piccinini [21]	RGB	X	X					X				X
Yuan [22]	RGB	X				X	X					X
Borges [23]	RGB					X					X	
Qi [24]	RGB/ HSV	X	X	X		X	X		X		X	
Yasmin [25]	RGB/ HSI									X		X
Gubbi [26]			X				X	X				X

State–of–the–art: underlying techniques (PART 3: 2010–2011).

Paper	Color detection	Moving object detection	Flicker/ energy (wavelet) analysis	Spatial difference analysis	Dynamic texture/ Pattern analysis	Disorder analysis	Subblocking	Training (models, NN, SVM, ...)	Cleanup post-processing	Localization/ analysis	Flame detection	Smoke detection
Chen [27]	RGB/ HSI	X	X					X			X	
Gunay [28]	RGB/ HSI	X	X	X		X		X			X	
Kolesov [29]		X			X			X			X	X
Ko [30]	RGB	X	X					X			X	
Gonzalez-Gonzalez [31]			X			X						X
Borges [32]	RGB			X	X	X		X			X	
Van Hamme [33]	HSV				X		X	X			X	
Celik [34]	CIE L*a*b*	X				X		X	X		X	
Yuan [35]					X			X	X			X
Rossi [36]	YUV/ RGB							X	X	X	X	

2.1.1 Color Detection

Color detection was one of the first detection techniques used in VFD and is still used in almost all detection methods. The majority of the color-based approaches in VFD make use of RGB color space, sometimes in combination with HSI/HSV saturation [10,24,27,28]. The main reason for using RGB is that almost all visible range cameras have sensors detecting video in RGB format and there is the obvious spectral content associated with this color space. It is reported that RGB values of flame pixels are in the red-yellow color range indicated by the rule (R > G > B) as shown in Fig. 2.1. Similarly, in smoke pixels, R, G, and B values are very close to each other. More complex systems use rule-based techniques such as Gaussian smoothed color histograms [7], statistically generated color models [15], and blending functions [20]. It is obvious that color cannot be used by itself to detect fire because of the variability in color, density, lighting, and background. However, the color information can be used as a part of a more sophisticated system. For example, chrominance decrease is used in smoke detection

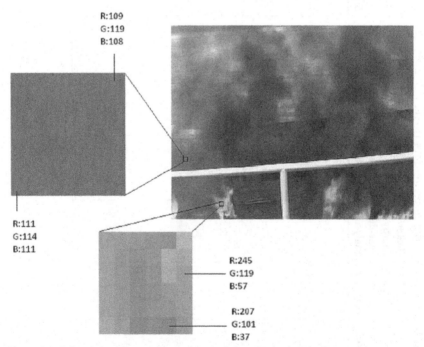

Figure 2.1 Color detection: smoke region pixels have color values that are close to each other. Pixels of flame regions lie in the red-yellow range of RGB color space with R > G > B.

schemes of Refs. [14,2]. Luminance value of smoke regions should be high for most smoke sources. On the other hand, the chrominance values should be very low.

The conditions in YUV color space are as follows:

Condition 1: $Y > T_Y$

Condition 2: $|U - 128| < T_U \, \& \, |V - 128| < T_V$.

where Y, U, and V are the luminance and chrominance values of a particular pixel, respectively. The luminance component Y takes values in the range $[0, 255]$ in an 8-bit quantized image and the mean values of chrominance channels U and V are increased to 128 so that they also take values between 0 and 255. The thresholds T_Y, T_U, and T_V are experimentally determined [37].

2.1.2 Moving Object Detection

Moving object detection is also widely used in VFD because flames and smoke are moving objects. To determine if the motion is due to smoke or an ordinary moving object, further analysis of moving regions in video is necessary.

Well-known moving object detection algorithms are background (BG) subtraction methods [16,21,18,14,13,17,20,22,27,28,30,34], temporal differencing [19], and optical flow analysis [9,8,29]. They can all be used as part of a VFD system.

In background subtraction methods, it is assumed that the camera is stationary. In Fig. 2.2, a background subtraction-based motion detection

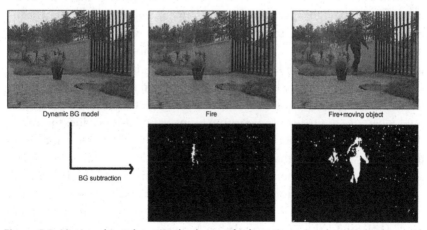

Figure 2.2 Moving object detection: background subtraction using dynamic background model.

example is shown using the dynamic background model proposed by Collins et al. [38]. This Gaussian Mixture Model-based approach model was used in many of the articles listed in tables above.

Some of the early VFD articles simply classified fire-colored moving objects as fire but this approach leads to many false alarms, because falling leaves in autumn or fire-colored ordinary objects, etc., may all be incorrectly classified as fire. Further analysis of motion in video is needed to achieve more accurate systems.

2.1.3 Motion and Flicker Analysis Using Fourier and Wavelet Transforms

As it is well known, flames flicker in uncontrolled fires, therefore flicker detection [24,18,12,13,27,28,30] in video and wavelet-domain signal energy analysis [21,14,20,26,31,39] can be used to distinguish ordinary objects from fire. These methods focus on the temporal behavior of flames and smoke. As a result, flame colored pixels appear and disappear at the edges of turbulent flames. The research in [16,18] shows experimentally that the flicker frequency of turbulent flames is around 10 Hz and that it is not greatly affected by the burning material and the burner. As a result, using frequency analysis to differentiate flames from other moving objects is proposed. However, an uncontrolled fire in its early stage exhibits a transition to chaos due to the fact that the combustion process consists of nonlinear instabilities which result in transition to chaotic behavior via intermittency [40–43]. Consequently, turbulent flames can be characterized as a chaotic wide-band frequency activity. Therefore, it is not possible to observe a single flickering frequency in the light spectrum due to an uncontrolled fire. This phenomenon was observed by independent researchers working on VFD and methods were proposed accordingly [14,44,27]. Similarly, it is not possible to talk about a specific flicker frequency for smoke, but we clearly observe a time-varying meandering behavior in uncontrolled fires. Therefore, smoke flicker detection does not seem to be a very reliable technique, but it can be used as part of a multi-feature algorithm fusing various vision clues for smoke detection. Temporal Fourier analysis can still be used to detect flickering flames, but we believe that there is no need to detect specifically 10 Hz. An increase in Fourier domain energy in 510 Hz is an indicator of flames.

The temporal behavior of smoke can be exploited by wavelet domain energy analysis. As smoke gradually softens the edges in an image, Toreyin et al. [14] found the energy variation between background and current image as a clue to detect the presence of smoke. In order to detect the energy decrease in edges of the image, they use the Discrete Wavelet Transform (DWT). The DWT is a multi-resolution signal decomposition method obtained by convolving the intensity image with filter banks. A standard halfband filterbank produces four wavelet subimages: the so-called low-low version of the original image C_t, and the horizontal, vertical, and diagonal high frequency band images H_t, V_t, and D_t. The high-band energy from subimages H_t, V_t, and D_t is evaluated by dividing the image I_t in blocks b_k of arbitrary size as follows:

$$E(I_t, b_k) = \sum_{i,j \in b_k} H_t^2(i,j) + V_t^2(i,j) + D_t^2(i,j) \qquad (2.1)$$

Since contribution of edges are more significant in highband wavelet images compared to flat areas of the image, it is possible to detect smoke using the decrease in $E(I_t, b_k)$. As the energy value of a specific block varies significantly over time in the presence of smoke, temporal analysis of the ratio between the current input frame wavelet energy and the background image wavelet energy is used to detect the smoke as shown in Fig. 2.3.

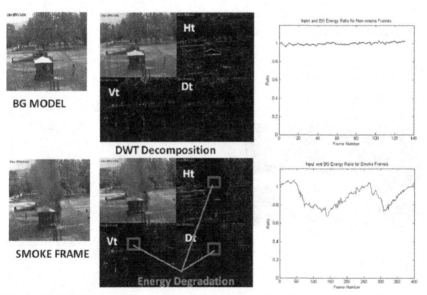

Figure 2.3 DWT-based video smoke detection: When there is smoke, the ratio between the input frame wavelet energy and the BG wavelet energy decreases and shows a high degree of disorder.

2.1.4 Spatial Wavelet Color Variation and Analysis

Flames of an uncontrolled fire have varying colors even within a small area. Spatial color difference analysis [24,13,28,32] focuses on this characteristic. Using range filters [24], variance/histogram analysis [32], or spatial wavelet analysis [13,28], the spatial color variations in pixel values are analyzed to distinguish ordinary fire-colored objects from uncontrolled fires. In Fig. 2.4, the concept of spatial difference analysis is further explained by means of a histogram-based approach, which focuses on the standard deviation of the green color band. It was observed by Qi and Ebert [24] that this color band is the most discriminative band for recognizing the spatial color variation of flames. This can also be seen by analyzing the histograms. Green pixel values vary more than red and blue values. If the standard deviation of the green color band exceeds $t_\sigma = 50$ (: Borges [32]) in a typical color video the region is labeled as a candidate region for a flame. For smoke detection, on the other hand, experiments revealed that these techniques are not always applicable because smoke regions often do not show as high spatial color variation as flame regions. Furthermore, textured smoke-colored moving objects are difficult to distinguish from smoke and can cause false detections. In general, smoke in an uncontrolled fire is gray and it reduces the color variation in the background. Therefore, in YUV color space we expect to have reduction in the dynamic range of chrominance color components U and V after the appearance of smoke in the viewing range of camera.

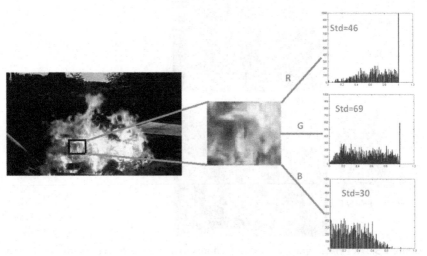

Figure 2.4 Spatial difference analysis: in case of flames, the standard deviation σ_G of the green color band of the flame region exceeds $t_\sigma = 50$ (: Borges [32]).

2.1.5 Dynamic Texture and Pattern Analysis

A dynamic texture or pattern in video, such as smoke, flames, water, and leaves in the wind, can be simply defined as a texture with motion [45,46] (ie, a spatially and time-varying visual pattern that forms an image sequence or part of an image sequence with a certain temporal stationarity) [47]. Although dynamic textures are easily observed by human eyes, they are difficult to discern using computer vision methods as the spatial location and extent of dynamic textures can vary with time and they can be partially transparent. Some dynamic texture and pattern analysis methods in video [29,33,35] are closely related to spatial difference analysis. Recently, these techniques have also been applied to the flame and smoke detection problem [46]. Currently, a wide variety of methods including geometric, model-based, statistical, and motion-based techniques are used for dynamic texture detection [48–50].

In Fig 2.5, dynamic texture detection and segmentation examples are shown, using video clips from the DynTex dynamic texture and Bilkent databases [51,52,50,47]. Contours of dynamic texture regions (eg, fire, water, and steam) are shown in this figure. Dynamic regions in video seem to be segmented very well. However, due to the high computational cost, these general techniques are not used in practical fire detection algorithms which should run on low-cost computers, FPGAs, or digital signal processors. If future developments in computers and graphics accelerators could lower the computational cost, dynamic texture detection methods may be incorporated into the currently available VFD systems to achieve more reliable systems.

Ordinary moving objects in video, such as walking people, have a pretty stable or almost periodic boundary over time. On the other hand, uncontrolled flame and smoke regions exhibit chaotic boundary contours. Therefore, disorder analysis of boundary contours of a moving object is useful for fire detection. Some examples of frequently used metrics are randomness of area size [23,32], boundary roughness [14,11,28,32], and boundary area

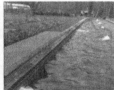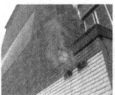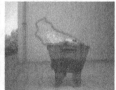

Figure 2.5 Dynamic texture detection: contours of detected dynamic texture regions are shown in the figure (*Results from DYNTEX and Bilkent databases* [51,53]).

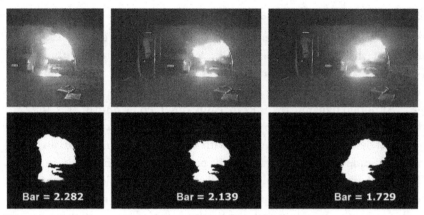

Figure 2.6 Boundary area roughness of consecutive flame regions.

disorder [18]. Although those metrics differ in definition, the outcome of each of them is almost identical. In the smoke detector developed by Verstock et al. [2], disorder analysis of the Boundary Area Roughness (BAR) is used, which is determined by relating the perimeter of the region to the square root of the area (Fig. 2.6). Another technique is the histogram-based orientation accumulation by Yuan [22]. This technique also produces good disorder detection results, but it is computationally more complex than the former methods. Related to the disorder analysis is the growing of smoke and flame regions in the early stage of a fire. In [31,34], the growth rate of the region-of-interest is used as a feature parameter for fire detection. Compared to disorder metrics, however, growth analysis is less effective in detecting the smoke, especially in wildfire detection. This is because the smoke region appears to grow very slowly in wildfires when they are viewed from long distances. Furthermore, an ordinary object may be approaching the camera.

2.2 SPATIOTEMPORAL NORMALIZED COVARIANCE DESCRIPTORS

A recent approach which combines color and spatiotemporal information by region covariance descriptors is used in European Commission funded FP-7 FIRESENSE project [54–56]. The method is based on analyzing the spatio-temporal blocks. The blocks are obtained by dividing the fire- and smoke-colored regions into 3D regions that overlap in time. Classification of the features is performed only at the temporal boundaries of blocks instead of performing it at each frame. This reduces the computational complexity of the method.

Covariance descriptors are proposed by Tuzel, Porikli, and Meer to be used in object detection and texture classification problems [54,55]. In [57,75,76] temporally extended normalized covariance descriptors to extract features from video sequences are proposed.

Temporally extended normalized covariance descriptors are designed to describe spatiotemporal video blocks. Let $I(i, j, n)$ be the intensity of (i, j)th pixel of the nth image frame of a spatiotemporal block in video. The property parameters defined in equations below are used to form a covariance matrix representing spatial information. In addition to spatial parameters, temporal derivatives, It and Itt are introduced which are the first and second derivatives of intensity with respect to time, respectively. By adding these two features to the previous property set, normalized covariance descriptors can be used to define spatiotemporal blocks in video.

For flame detection:

$$R_{i,j,n} = Red(i, j, n), \tag{2.2}$$

$$G_{i,j,n} = Green(i, j, n), \tag{2.3}$$

$$B_{i,j,n} = Blue(i, j, n), \tag{2.4}$$

$$I_{i,j,n} = Intensity(i, j, n), \tag{2.5}$$

$$Ix_{i,j,n} = \left| \frac{\partial Intensity(i, j, n)}{\partial i} \right|, \tag{2.6}$$

$$Iy_{i,j,n} = \left| \frac{\partial Intensity(i, j, n)}{\partial j} \right|, \tag{2.7}$$

$$Ixx_{i,j,n} = \left| \frac{\partial^2 Intensity(i, j, n)}{\partial i^2} \right|, \tag{2.8}$$

$$Iyy_{i,j,n} = \left| \frac{\partial^2 Intensity(i, j, n)}{\partial j^2} \right|, \tag{2.9}$$

$$It_{i,j,n} = \left| \frac{\partial Intensity(i, j, n)}{\partial n} \right|, \tag{2.10}$$

$$\text{and } Itt_{i,j,n} = \left| \frac{\partial^2 Intensity(i, j, n)}{\partial n^2} \right| \tag{2.11}$$

For smoke detection:

$$Y_{i,j,n} = Luminance(i,j,n), \tag{2.12}$$

$$U_{i,j,n} = ChrominanceU(i,j,n), \tag{2.13}$$

$$V_{i,j,n} = ChrominanceV(i,j,n), \tag{2.14}$$

$$I_{i,j,n} = Intensity(i,j,n), \tag{2.15}$$

$$Ix_{i,j,n} = \left| \frac{\partial Intensity(i,j,n)}{\partial i} \right|, \tag{2.16}$$

$$Iy_{i,j,n} = \left| \frac{\partial Intensity(i,j,n)}{\partial j} \right|, \tag{2.17}$$

$$Ixx_{i,j,n} = \left| \frac{\partial^2 Intensity(i,j,n)}{\partial i^2} \right|, \tag{2.18}$$

$$Iyy_{i,j,n} = \left| \frac{\partial^2 Intensity(i,j,n)}{\partial j^2} \right|, \tag{2.19}$$

$$It_{i,j,n} = \left| \frac{\partial Intensity(i,j,n)}{\partial n} \right|, \tag{2.20}$$

$$Itt_{i,j,n} = \left| \frac{\partial^2 Intensity(i,j,n)}{\partial n^2} \right| \tag{2.21}$$

In order to improve the detection performance, the majority of the articles in the literature use a combination of the fire feature extraction methods described above. Depending on the fire/environmental characteristics, one combination of features will outperform the other, and vice versa. In Section 2.4, we describe an adaptive fusion method combining the results of various fire detection methods in an online manner.

It should be pointed out that articles in the literature and those which are referenced in this state-of-the-art review indicate that ordinary visible range camera-based detection systems promise good fire detection results. However, they still suffer from a significant amount of missed detections and false alarms in practical situations, as in other computer vision problems [5,6]. The main cause of these problems is the fact that visual detection is often subject to constraints regarding the scene under investigation (eg, changing environmental conditions, different camera parameters, and color settings and illumination). It is also impossible to compare the articles with each other and determine the best one. This is because they use different training and data sets.

A data set of fire and non-fire videos is available to the research community in European Commission funded FIRESENSE project web page [56]. These test videos were used for training and testing purposes of the smoke and flame detection algorithms developed within the FIRESENSE project. Thus, a fair comparison of the algorithms developed by individual partners could be conducted. The test database includes 27 test and 29 training sequences of visible spectrum recordings of flame scenes, 15 test and 27 training sequences of visible spectrum recordings of smoke scenes, and 22 test and 27 training sequences of visible spectrum recordings of forest smoke scenes. This database is currently available to registered users of the FIRESENSE website [Reference: FIRESENSE project File Repository, http://www.firesense.eu, 2012].

2.3 CLASSIFICATION TECHNIQUES

A popular approach for the classification of the multi-dimensional feature vectors obtained from each candidate flame or smoke blob is SVM classification, typically with Radial Basis Function (RBF) kernels. A large number of frames of fire and non-fire video sequences need to be used for training these SVM classifiers; otherwise the number of false alarms (false positives or true negatives) may be significantly increased.

Other classification methods include the AdaBoost method [22], neural networks [29,35], Bayesian classifiers [30,32], Markov models [28,33], and rule-based classification [58].

As in any video processing method, morphological operations, sub-blocking, and clean-up post-processing, such as median-filtering, are used as an integral part of any VFD system [21,22,25,20,26,33,36,59].

2.4 EVALUATION OF VISIBLE RANGE VFD METHODS

An evaluation of different visible range VFD methods is presented in Table 2.1. Table 2.1 summarizes comparative detection results for the smoke and flame detection algorithm by Verstockt [2] (Method 1), a combination of the flame detection method by Celik et al. [60] and the smoke detection by Toreyin et al. [14] (Method 2) and a combination of the feature-based flame detection method by Borges et al. [23] and the smoke detection method by Xiong et al. [18] (Method 3). Among various algorithms, Verstockt's method is a relatively recent one, whereas flame detection methods by Celik and Borges and the smoke detection methods by Toreyin and Xiong are commonly referenced methods in the literature.

Table 2.1 An evaluation of different visible range VFD methods

Video sequence (# frames)	# Fire frames ground truth	# Detected fire frames			# False positive frames			Detection rate*		
		Method			Method			Method		
		1	2	3	1	2	3	1	2	3
Paper fire (1550)	956	897	922	874	9	17	22	0.93	0.95	0.89
Car fire (2043)	1415	1293	1224	1037	3	8	13	0.91	0.86	0.73
Moving people (886)	0	5	0	28	5	0	28	–	–	–
Wood fire (592)	522	510	489	504	17	9	16	0.94	0.92	0.93
Bunsen burner (115)	98	59	53	32	0	0	0	0.60	0.54	0.34
Moving car (332)	0	0	13	11	0	13	11	–	–	–
Straw fire (938)	721	679	698	673	16	21	12	0.92	0.93	0.92
Smoke/fog machine (1733)	923	834	654	789	9	34	52	0.89	0.67	0.80
Pool fire (2260)	1844	1665	1634	1618	0	0	0	0.90	0.89	0.88

*Detection rate = (# detected fire frames − # false alarms)/# fire frames.

Test sequences used for performance evaluation are captured in different environments under various conditions. Snapshots from test videos are presented in Fig. 2.7. In order to objectively evaluate the detection results of different methods, the "detection rate" metric [2,61] is used, which is comparable to the evaluation methods used by Celik et al. [60] and Toreyin et al. [13]. The detection rate equals the ratio of the number of correctly detected frames as fire (ie, the detected frames as fire minus the number of falsely detected frames) to the number of frames with fire in the manually created ground truth frames. As results indicate, the detection performances of different methods are comparable with each other.

Comparison of the smoke and flame detection method by Verstockt [2] (Method 1), the combined method based on the flame detector by Celik et al. [60] and the smoke detector described in Toreyin et al. [14] (Method 2), and combination of the feature–based flame detection method by Borges et al. [23] and the smoke detection method by Xiong et al. [18] (Method 3).

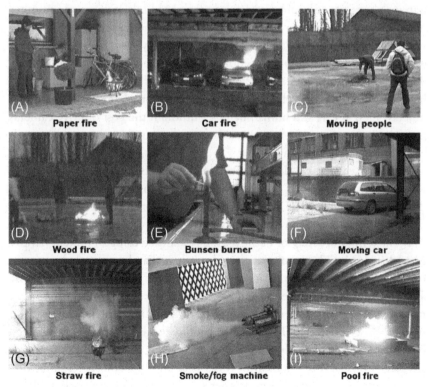

Figure 2.7 Snapshots from test sequences with and without fire.

2.5 VFD IN IR SPECTRAL RANGE

When there is very little or no visible light, or the color of the object to be detected is similar to the background, IR imaging systems provide solutions [62–68]. Although there is an increasing trend in IR camera-based intelligent video analysis, there are very few papers in the area of IR-based fire detection [64–68]. This is mainly due to the high cost of IR imaging systems compared to ordinary cameras. Manufacturers predict that IR camera prices will go down in the near future. Therefore, we expect that the number of IR imaging applications will increase significantly [63]. Long-wave Infrared (8-12 micron range) cameras are the most widely available cameras on the market. Long-wave Infrared (LWIR) light goes through smoke, therefore it is easy to detect smoke using LWIR imaging systems. Nevertheless, results from existing work already ensure the feasibility of IR cameras for flame detection.

Owrutsky et al. [64] worked in the NIR spectral range and compared the global luminosity L, which is the sum of the pixel intensities of the current frame, to a reference luminosity L_b and a threshold Lth. If there are a number of consecutive frames where L exceeds the persistence criterion $L_b + Lth$, the system goes into an alarm stage. Although this fairly simple algorithm seems to produce good results in the reported experiments, its limited constraints do raise questions about its applicability in large and open uncontrolled public places and it will probably produce many false alarms to hot moving objects, such as cars and human beings. Although the cost of NIR cameras is not high, their imaging ranges are shorter compared to visible range cameras and other IR cameras.

Toreyin et al. [65] detect flames in LWIR by searching for bright-looking moving objects with rapid time-varying contours. A wavelet domain analysis of the 1D-curve representation of the contours is used to detect the high frequency nature of the boundary of a fire region. In addition, the temporal behavior of the region is analyzed using a Hidden Markov Model (HMM). The combination of both spatial and temporal clues seems more appropriate than the luminosity approach and, according to the authors their approach greatly reduces false alarms caused by ordinary bright moving objects. A similar combination of temporal and spatial features is also used by Bosch et al. [66]. Hotspots (ie, candidate flame regions) are detected by automatic histogram-based image thresholding. By analyzing the intensity, signature, and orientation of these resulting hot objects' regions, discrimination between flames and other objects is made. Verstock et al. [2]

also proposed an IR-based fire detector which mainly follows the latter feature-based strategy, but contrary to Bosch et al.'s work [66] a dynamic background subtraction method is used, which aims at coping with the time-varying characteristics of dynamic scenes.

To sum up, it should be pointed out that it is not straightforward to detect fires using IR cameras. Not every bright object in IR video is a source of wildfire. It is important to mention that IR imaging has its own specific limitations, such as thermal reflections, IR blocking, and thermal-distance problems. In some situations, IR-based detection will perform better than visible VFD, but under other circumstances, visible VFD can improve IR flame detection. This is due to the fact that smoke appears earlier and becomes visible from long distances in a typical uncontrolled fire. Flames and burning objects may not be in the viewing range of the IR camera. As such, higher detection accuracies with lower false alarm rates can be achieved by combining multi-spectrum video information. Various image fusion methods may be employed for this purpose [69,70]. Clearly, each sensor type has its own specific limitations, which can only be compensated by other types of sensors.

2.6 WILDFIRE SMOKE DETECTION USING VISIBLE RANGE CAMERAS

As pointed out in the previous section, smoke is clearly visible from long distances in wildfires and forest fires. In most cases, flames are hindered by trees. Therefore, IR imaging systems may not provide solutions for early fire detection in wildfires but ordinary visible range cameras can detect smoke from long distances.

There are many methods in the literature for wildfire smoke detection [37,71,77]. The method developed for FIRESENSE [56] project combines rule-based and learning-based methods. There are five main algorithms used in the method.

The first algorithm uses double IIR-based background subtraction and double backgrounds to find slow-moving regions. During the initial phases of wildfire, smoke appears to move slowly when viewed from a distance. This observation is used to separate slow moving smoke regions from other fast moving objects.

The second algorithm uses thresholds in YUV color space to extract smoke colored regions. Smoke is assumed to have gray-to-white color during the initial stages of wildfire caused by the burning of vegetation.

The third algorithm uses DWT to classify smooth regions. The scenes in wildfire scenarios usually contain high-pass elements consisting of trees, rocks, and terrain. When smoke appears, it can smooth the edges of the current image compared to the background. This phenomenon is quantified using the ratio of the wavelet energies of background and foreground images.

The fourth algorithm tries to eliminate false alarms caused by moving cloud shadows. The angles of RGB color channels between the background and foreground images are used to decide if a moving region is cloud shadow.

The fifth algorithm uses covariance matrix-based feature extraction and support vector machine (SVM) classification. Features are extracted from smoke-colored moving regions and are fed to the SVM classifier.

The most important problem with video-based wildfire detection systems is the high number of false alarms caused by dynamic environments. In [37,71,77], online classifier fusion methods are proposed to adaptively combine the previously described algorithms. Different methods can be used to combine different algorithms. Orthogonal and entropic projections onto convex are some of the proposed supervised learning methods. The weights of the algorithms are adjusted online using the supervision of the security guard at the watch tower. Whenever there is a false alarm, the guard can mark it as a false positive and the weights are updated accordingly.

If we M algorithms with outputs, $\mathbf{x}_t = [\mathbf{x}_t(1),\ldots,\mathbf{x}_t(M)]^T$, at time step t. We denote the weights of classifiers as $\mathbf{w}_t = [\mathbf{w}_t(1),\ldots,\mathbf{w}_t(M)]^T$. The output of the linear combination can be written as follows:

$$\hat{y}_t = x_t^T w = \sum_i w_t(i) x_t(i)$$

This is an estimate of the true binary class label y_t. The error is also defined as $e_t = y_t - \hat{y}_t$.

When orthogonal projections are used, the weights are updated as follows:

$$\mathbf{w}_{t+1} = \mathbf{w}_t + \frac{e_t}{\|\mathbf{x}_t\|_2^2} \mathbf{x}_t.$$

Most wildfire detections systems use PTZ cameras that move between predefined positions and run the detection algorithms while the camera is stationary. In the online classifier fusion methods, separate weights are assigned to each position and they are updated independently to achieve faster convergence.

2.7 WILDFIRE DETECTION FROM MOVING AERIAL PLATFORMS

Cameras installed on unmanned aerial vehicles (UAVs) or aircrafts can be used increase coverage area for early detection of wildfires. Since the platform is always in motion and the environment changes constantly, online learning algorithms can be used to reduce false alarms for this detection method.

Traditional wildfire detection systems first detect slow-moving regions with stationary cameras and then use rule- or learning-based algorithms to decide existence of smoke. Since aerial platforms are in motion, it is difficult to extract moving smoke regions. Therefore in this section, a wildfire detection system is described that does not use motion information. First the whole image is segmented using a segmentation algorithm that can distinguish smoke regions as a separate segment. Then features are extracted from the segments that satisfy certain criteria. The features are classified using online learning algorithms.

A graph-based image segmentation method is used to segment smoke regions. This method can maintain detail in low-pass regions and discard detail in high-pass regions. This helps the algorithm to segment smoke regions which have low-frequency characteristics compared to the forest terrain. In Fig. 2.8, segmentation result of a real wildfire is displayed that is recorded from a helicopter.

Color analysis of candidate segments is performed to find smoke-colored regions. Wildfire smoke usually has gray-to-white color in early stages. Thresholds in YUV color space are used to check color content of segments.

Features are extracted from the segments that satisfy color condition. The features represent the color, texture, and shape characteristics of regions. RGB histograms are used to form color features. Dual-tree complex wavelet

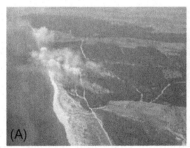
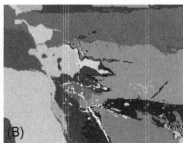

Figure 2.8 Segmentation results for helicopter images.

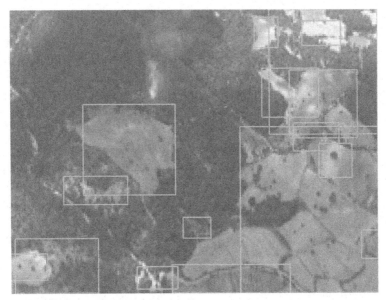

Figure 2.9 Wildfire smoke detection results.

transform (DT-CWT) is used to form texture features [72]. Zernike moments are used to extract shape features [73].

Online binary classification algorithms learn the weights of each feature element in real time with user supervision. Passive aggressive (PA) method is a maximum-margin algorithm that maximizes the margin defined by $y_t(w_t \cdot x_t)$, where y_t is the label, w_t is the weight vector, x_t is the feature vector [74]. The procedure used to update the weight vector depends on the specific application.

Fig. 2.9 shows sample wildfire detection results. The bounding boxes of segments are marked with rectangles and the segments classified as smoke are marked red.

REFERENCES

[1] A.E. Çetin, K. Dimitropoulos, B. Gouverneur, N. Grammalidis, O. Günay, Y. Hakan Habiboğlu, B. Uğur Töreyin, S. Verstockt, Video fire detection—Review, Digital Signal Process. 1051-2004, 23 (6) (2013) 1827–1843.
[2] S. Verstockt, Multi-modal video analysis for early fire detection, Ph.D. Thesis, Universiteit Gent, 2011.
[3] H.L. Dreyfus, What Computers Can't Do, MIT Press, Cambridge, MA, 1972.
[4] H.L. Dreyfus, What Computers Still Can't Do, MIT Press, Cambridge, MA, 1992.
[5] T. Pavlidis, Computers versus humans, http://www.theopavlidis.com/comphumans/comphuman.htm.

[6] T. Pavlidis, Why machine intelligence is so hard—a discussion of the difference between human and computer intelligence, http://www.theopavlidis.com/technology/MachineIntel/index.htm.

[7] W. Phillips, M. Shah, N. da Vitoria Lobo, Flame recognition in video, Pattern Recogn. Lett. 23 (1–3) (2002) 319–327.

[8] F. Gomez-Rodriguez, S. Pascual-Pena, B. Arrue, A. Ollero, Smoke detection using image processing, in: Proceedings of 4th International Conference on Forest Fire Research & Wildland Fire Safety, 2002, pp. 1–8.

[9] F. Gomez-Rodriguez, B.C. Arrue, A. Ollero, Smoke monitoring and measurement using image processing—application to forest fires, in: Proceedings of SPIE AeroSense 2003: XIII Automatic Target Recognition, 2003, pp. 404–411.

[10] T.-H. Chen, P.-H. Wu, Y.-C. Chiou, An early fire-detection method based on image processing, in: Proceedings of IEEE International Conference on Image Processing (ICIP), vol. 3, 2004, pp. 1707–1710.

[11] C.B. Liu, N. Ahuja, Vision based fire detection, in: Proceedings of 17th International Conference on Pattern Recognition (ICPR), vol. 4, 2004, pp. 134–137.

[12] G. Marbach, M. Loepfe, T. Brupbacher, An image processing technique for fire detection in video images, Fire Saf. J. 41 (4) (2006) 285–289.

[13] B.U. Toreyin, Y. Dedeoglu, U. Gudukbay, A.E. Cetin, Computer vision based method for real-time fire and flame detection, Pattern Recogn. Lett. 27 (1) (2006) 49–58.

[14] B.U. Toreyin, Y. Dedeoglu, A.E. Cetin, Contour based smoke detection in video using wavelets, in: Proceedings of European Signal Processing Conference (EUSIPCO), 2006.

[15] T. Celik, H. Ozkaramanli, H. Demirel, Fire and smoke detection without sensors: image processing based approach, in: Proceedings of 15th European Signal Processing Conference (EUSIPCO), 2007, pp. 1794–1798.

[16] Z. Xu, J. Xu, Automatic fire smoke detection based on image visual features, in: Proceedings of International Conference on Computational Intelligence and Security Workshops, 2007, pp. 316–319.

[17] T. Celik, H. Demirel, H. Ozkaramanli, M. Uyguroglu, Fire detection using statistical color model in video sequences, J. Vis. Commun. Image Represent. 18 (2) (2007) 176–185.

[18] Z. Xiong, R. Caballero, H. Wang, A.M. Finn, M.A. Lelic, P.-Y. Peng, Video-based smoke detection: possibilities, techniques, and challenges, in: Proceedings of Suppression and Detection Research and Applications (SUPDET)—A Technical Working Conference, 2007.

[19] B. Lee, D. Han, Real-time fire detection using camera sequence image in tunnel environment, in: Proceedings of International Conference on Intelligent, Computing, 2007, pp. 1209–1220.

[20] S. Calderara, P. Piccinini, V. Cucchiara, Smoke detection in video surveillance: a MoG model in the wavelet domain, in: Proceedings of 6th International Conference in Computer Vision Systems (ICVS), 2008, pp. 119–128.

[21] P. Piccinini, S. Calderara, R. Cucchiara, Reliable smoke detection system in the domains of image energy and color, in: Proceedings of International Conference on Image Processing, 2008, pp. 1376–1379.

[22] F. Yuan, A fast accumulative motion orientation model based on integral image for video smoke detection, Pattern Recogn. Lett. 29 (7) (2008) 925–932.

[23] P.V.K. Borges, J. Mayer, E. Izquierdo, Efficient visual fire detection applied for video retrieval, in: Proceedings of 16th European Signal Processing Conference (EUSIPCO), 2008.

[24] X. Qi, J. Ebert, A computer vision based method for fire detection in color videos, Int. J. Imag. 2 (S09) (2009) 22–34. Spring.

[25] R. Yasmin, Detection of smoke propagation direction using color video sequences, Int. J. Soft Comput. 4 (1) (2009) 45–48.

[26] J. Gubbi, S. Marusic, M. Palaniswami, Smoke detection in video using wavelets and support vector machines, Fire Saf. J. 44 (8) (2009) 1110–1115.

[27] J. Chen, Y. He, J. Wang, Multi-feature fusion based fast video flame detection, Build. Environ. 45 (5) (2010) 1113–1122.

[28] O. Gunay, K. Tasdemir, B.U. Töreyin, A.E. Cetin, Fire detection in video using lms based active learning, Fire. Technol 46 (3) (2010) 551–577.

[29] I. Kolesov, P. Karasev, A. Tannenbaum, E. Haber, Fire and smoke detection in video with optimal mass transport based optical flow and neural networks, in: Proceedings of IEEE International Conference on Image Processing (ICIP), 2010, pp. 761–764.

[30] B.C. Ko, K.H. Cheong, J.Y. Nam, Early fire detection algorithm based on irregular patterns of flames and hierarchical Bayesian networks, Fire Saf. J. 45 (4) (2010) 262–270.

[31] R.A. Gonzalez-Gonzalez, V. Alarcon-Aquino, O. Starostenko, R. Rosas-Romero, J.M. Ramirez-Cortes, J. Rodriguez-Asomoza, Wavelet-based smoke detection in outdoor video sequences, in: Proceedings of the 53rd IEEE Midwest Symposium on Circuits and Systems (MWSCAS), 2010, pp. 383–387.

[32] P.V.K. Borges, E. Izquierdo, A probabilistic approach for vision-based fire detection in videos, IEEE Trans. Circuits Syst. Video Technol. 20 (5) (2010) 721–731.

[33] D. Van Hamme, P. Veelaert, W. Philips, K. Teelen, Fire detection in color images using Markov random fields, in: Proceedings of Advanced Concepts for Intelligent Vision Systems (ACIVS), vol. 2, 2010, pp. 88–97.

[34] T. Celik, Fast and efficient method for fire detection using image processing, ETRI J. 32 (6) (2010) 881–890.

[35] F. Yuan, Video-based smoke detection with histogram sequence of lbp and lbpv pyramids, Fire Saf. J. 46 (3) (2011) 132–139.

[36] L. Rossi, M. Akhloufi, Y. Tison, On the use of stereo vision to develop a novel instrumentation system to extract geometric fire fronts characteristics, Fire Saf. J. (Forest Fires) 46 (1–2) (2011) 9–20.

[37] B.U. Töreyin, Fire detection algorithms using multimodal signal and image analysis, Ph.D. Thesis, Bilkent University, 2009.

[38] R.T. Collins, A.J. Lipton, T. Kanade, A system for video surveillance and monitoring, in: Proceedings of American Nuclear Society (ANS) Eighth International Topical Meeting on Robotics and Remote Systems, 1999.

[39] S. Calderara, P. Piccinini, R. Cucchiara, Vision based smoke detection system using image energy and color information, Mach. Vis. Appl. 22 (4) (2010) 705–719.

[40] M. Wendeker, J. Czarnigowski, G. Litak, K. Szabelski, Chaotic Combustion in spark ignition engines, Chaos, Solitons and Fractals 18 (2004) 805–808.

[41] P. Manneville, Instabilities, Chaos and Turbulence, Imperial College Press, London, 2004.

[42] C.K. Law, Combustion Physics, Cambridge University Press, New York, 2006.

[43] V. Gubernov, A. Kolobov, A. Polezhaev, H. Sidhu, G. Mercer, Period doubling and chaotic transient in a model of chain-branching combustion wave propagation, Proc. R. Soc. A 466 (2121) (2010) 2747–2769.

[44] J. Yang, R.S. Wang, A survey on fire detection and application based on video image analysis, Video Eng. 2006 (8) (2006) 92–96.

[45] G. Doretto, A. Chiuso, Y.N. Wu, S. Soatto, Dynamic textures, Int. J. Comput. Vis. 51 (2) (2003) 91–109.

[46] F. Porikli, A.E. Cetin, Special issue on dynamic textures in video, Mach. Vis. Appl. 22 (5) (2011) 739–740.

[47] T. Amiaz, S. Fazekas, D. Chetverikov, N. Kiryati, Detecting regions of dynamic texture, in: Proceedings of International Conference on Scale-Space and variational methods in Computer Vision (SSVM), 2007, pp. 848–859.

[48] D. Chetverikov, R. Peteri, D. Chetverikov, R. Peteri, A brief survey of dynamic texture description and recognition, in: Proceedings of 4th International Conference on Computer Recognition Systems, 2005, pp. 17–26.

[49] B.U. Toreyin, Y. Dedeoglu, A.E. Cetin, S. Fazekas, D. Chetverikov, T. Amiaz, N. Kiryati, Dynamic texture detection, segmentation and analysis, in: Proceedings of ACM International Conference on Image and Video Retrieval (CIVR), 2007, pp. 131–134.

[50] S. Fazekas, T. Amiaz, D. Chetverikov, N. Kiryati, Dynamic texture detection based on motion analysis, Int. J. Comput. Vis. 82 (1) (2009) 48–63.

[51] R. Péteri, S. Fazekas, M.J. Huiskes, DynTex: a comprehensive database of dynamic textures. Pattern Recogn. Lett. 31 (12) (2010) 1627–1632, http://dx.doi.org/10.1016/j.patrec.2010.05.009.

[52] S. Fazekas, D. Chetverikov, Analysis and performance evaluation of optical flow features for dynamic texture recognition, Signal Process. 22 (7–8) (2007) 680–691.

[53] A.E. Cetin, Computer vision based fire detection software—sample video clips, http://signal.ee.bilkent.edu.tr/VisiFire/.

[54] O. Tuzel, F. Porikli, P. Meer, Region covariance: A fast descriptor for detection and classification, in: Computer Vision—ECCV 2006, 2006, pp. 589–600.

[55] H. Tuna, I. Onaran, A.E. Çetin, Image description using a multiplier-less operator, IEEE Signal Process. Lett. 16 (9) (2009) 751–753.

[56] FIRESENSE, Fire detection and management through a multi-sensor network for the protection of cultural heritage areas from the risk of fire and extreme weather conditions, fp7-env-2009-1-244088-firesense, (2009). http://www.firesense.eu.

[57] Y. Habiboglu, O. Gunay, A.E. Cetin, Flame detection method in video using covariance descriptors, in: Acoustics, Speech and Signal Processing (ICASSP), 2011 IEEE International Conference on, 2011, 2011, pp. 1817–1820.

[58] Fire Safety Engineering (Bart Merci), Fire Safety and Explosion Safety in Car Parks.

[59] Y. Dedeoglu, B.U. Töreyin, U. Güdükbay, A.E. Çetin, Real-time fire and flame detection in video, in: International Conference on Acoustics Speech and Signal Processing (ICASSP), 2005, pp. 669–672.

[60] T. Celik, H. Demirel, Fire detection in video sequences using a generic color model, Fire Saf. J. 44 (2) (2008) 147–158.

[61] S. Verstockt, A. Vanoosthuyse, S. Van Hoecke, P. Lambert, R. Van de Walle, Multisensor fire detection by fusing visual and non-visual flame features, in: Proceedings of International Conference on Image and, Signal Processing, 2010, pp. 333–341.

[62] J. Han, B. Bhanu, Fusion of color and infrared video for moving human detection, Pattern Recogn. 40 (6) (2007) 1771–1784.

[63] R. Vandersmissen, Night-vision camera combines thermal and low-light-level images, Photonik Int. 2008 (2) (2008) 2–4.

[64] J.C. Owrutsky, D.A. Steinhurst, C.P. Minor, S.L. Rose-Pehrsson, F.W. Williams, D.T. Gottuk, Long wavelength video detection of fire in ship compartments, Fire Saf. J. 41 (4) (2006) 315–320.

[65] B.U. Toreyin, R.G. Cinbis, Y. Dedeoglu, A.E. Cetin, Fire detection in infrared video using wavelet analysis, SPIE Opt. Eng. 46 (6) (2007) 1–9.

[66] I. Bosch, S. Gomez, R. Molina, R. Miralles, Object discrimination by infrared image processing, in: Proceedings of the 3rd International Work-Conference on The Interplay Between Natural and Artificial Computation (IWINAC), 2009, pp. 30–40.

[67] O. Gunay, K. Tasdemir, B.U. Töreyin, A.E. Cetin, Video based wildfire detection at night, Fire Saf. J. 44 (6) (2009) 860–868.

[68] S. Verstockt, R. Dekeerschieter, A. Vanoosthuyse, B. Merci, B. Sette, P. Lambert, R. Van de Walle, Video fire detection using non-visible light, in: Proceedings of the 6th International Seminar on Fire and Explosion Hazards, 2010.

[69] V. Bruni, D. Vitulano, Z. Wang, Special issue on human vision and information theory, SIViP 7 (3) (2013) 389–390.

[70] S. Roy, T. Howlader, S.M. Mahbubur Rahman, Image fusion technique using multivariate statistical model for wavelet coefficients, SIViP 7 (2) (2013) 355–365.

[71] O. Gunay, B.U. Toreyin, K. Kose, A.E. Cetin, Entropy-functional-based online adaptive decision fusion framework with application to wildfire detection in video, IEEE Trans. Image Process. 21 (5) (2012) 2853–2865.

[72] I.W. Selesnick, R.G. Baraniuk, N.C. Kingsbury, The dual-tree complex wavelet transform, IEEE Signal Process. Mag. 22 (6) (2005) 123–151.

[73] A. Tahmasbi, F. Saki, S.B. Shokouhi, Classification of benign and malignant masses based on Zernike moments, Comput. Biol. Med. 41 (8) (2011) 726–735.

[74] K. Crammer, O. Dekel, J. Keshet, S. Shalev-Shwartz, Y. Singer, Online passive-aggressive algorithms, J. Mach. Learn. Res. 7 (2006) 551–585.

[75] Y.H. Habiboğlu, O. Günay, A.E. Çetin, Covariance matrix-based fire and flame detection method in video, Mach. Vis. Appl. 23 (6) (2012) 1103–1113.

[76] Y.H. Habiboglu, O. Gunay, A.E. Cetin, Real-time wildfire detection using correlation descriptors, in: 19th European Signal Processing Conference (EUSIPCO 2011), 2011.

[77] O. Gunay, Video processing algorithms for wildfire surveillance, Ph.D. Thesis, Bilkent University, 2015.

Part 2

2.8 WILDFIRE DETECTION WITH PTZ CAMERAS USING PANORAMIC BACKGROUNDS

In this part, we describe a real-time panoramic background estimation method for fast wildfire detection using continuously moving cameras [22]. Panoramic background generation has many uses for image processing and surveillance applications. Panoramic background generation mainly depends on efficient registration of successive images in the panoramic sequence. Registration algorithms can either be feature-based [1] or global [2]. Feature-based methods try to match the locations of features between the images, whereas global methods optimize a similarity measure to find a transformation matrix that best matches the images.

In [3], a real-time method for image to panorama registration is proposed. When forming the panorama, they also generate a set of key frames and during the real-time registration process they register each new image to the closest key frame. In this way, they overcome the error accumulation problem that can result from successive registrations to the panorama.

In [4], they use scale invariant feature transform (SIFT) and dynamic programming. SIFT is used for feature extraction and dynamic programming is used to stitch the panorama without artifacts. There are many other methods for panoramic image generation and its applications [5–12], but the key-frame-based method has the highest potential for the wildfire detection problem.

In our system, we consider continuously moving cameras for early detection of wildfires. Current wide area wildfire detection camera systems scan predefined preset positions and run the detection algorithm suited to stationary cameras. This can increase the detection time substantially when full 360-degree coverage of the area is needed. Therefore, we propose a wildfire detection system using continuously moving cameras. We use a hybrid registration method employing speeded-up robust features (SURF) and mutual information (MI) to form the panoramic background and select the keyframes. In the normal mode, we use SURF for matching each image to the previous frame; when the number of inliers between the images is not enough, we use mutual information-based optimization to find the transformation matrix. In the real-time operating mode, we again use a mutual information-based similarity measure to match the current image to one of the key frames. We then update the key frames that correspond to the background using the matched section of the current image.

After finding the moving regions, we track them and form a spatiotemporal video block that falls into the same region of the key frame. We then extract features from this block using local binary patterns (LBPs). We feed the features to a support vector machine to decide if the block belongs to a wildfire region.

2.8.1 Panorama Generation

2.8.1.1 Robust Features

We use SURF for feature extraction and matching. Random samples consensus (RANSAC) is used for finding the homography between a pair of images. After finding the homography matrix, we warp one of the images using a projective transform and add the next image to overlap the matching features. SIFT features are extracted around interest points and they can be used to match descriptors across different views of an image [1]. They are invariant to orientation and scale and they are robust to most affine viewpoint changes, different illuminations, and noise. The first step in SIFT feature extraction is the generation of Gaussian and difference of Gaussian (DOG) pyramids. The candidate keypoints are determined by finding the local maximum/minimum of the DOG images. After removing unstable keypoints, an orientation and a scale are assigned to each of the remaining keypoints. The orientations of the pixels around the keypoint are used to create an orientation histogram. SIFT method is computationally costly and therefore SURF method is generally preferred in real-time applications. SURF uses integral images for convolutions and Haar wavelets for features [13].

2.8.1.2 Mutual Information

We optimize a mutual information-based cost function to correctly register images when SURF method fails to find any inliers. For two random variables A and B, the MI measures the degree of dependence between the random variables and is defined as follows:

$$\text{MI}(A, B) = H(A) + H(B) - H(A, B) \qquad (2.22)$$

where $H(A)$, $H(B)$ are marginal entropies and $H(A,B)$ is the joint entropy. In image registration problems entropy functions are estimated from image histograms and joint histograms which can be calculated using kernel density estimation methods [2]. Shannon entropy of a discrete random variable can be defined as follows:

$$H(A) = -\sum_x p_A(x) \log(p_A(x)) \tag{2.23}$$

For image registration we first need to estimate the probabilistic distribution of the pixel values of images:

$$p_A(z) = \frac{1}{N} \sum_x R(z - A(x)) \tag{2.24}$$

where N denotes the number of samples that are used for the density estimation. In the usual histogram estimation R is the Kronecker delta function, and in kernel density applications R is a kernel such as Gaussian or B-spline functions. Joint density for two random variables can be also estimated as follows:

$$p_{A,B}(z, r) = \frac{1}{N} \sum_x R(z - A(x)) R(r - B(x)) \tag{2.25}$$

Using the density estimates, MI for images can be approximated as follows [2]:

$$\begin{aligned}
\text{MI}(I_V, I_R) \approx &\frac{-1}{N_B} \left\{ \sum_{I_V(i) \in B} \ln \frac{1}{N_A} \sum_{I_V(j) \in A} R(I_V(i) - I_V(j)) \right\} \\
&+ \frac{-1}{N_B} \left\{ \sum_{I_R(i) \in B} \ln \frac{1}{N_A} \sum_{I_R(j) \in A} R(I_R(i) - I_R(j)) \right\} \\
&- \frac{-1}{N_B} \left\{ \sum_{I_W(i) \in B} \ln \frac{1}{N_A} \sum_{I_W(j) \in A} R(I_W(i) - I_W(j)) \right\}
\end{aligned} \tag{2.26}$$

where R is the Gaussian window used in kernel density estimation, $I_W(i) = [I_V(i) \ I_R(i)]$. N_A and N_B denote the sizes of different sample sets. For optimization of the MI cost function various methods can be used, gradient descent, quasi-Newton or genetic algorithms are standard choices.

2.8.1.3 Finding Key Frames

We use a projective transformation matrix that has eight unknowns:

$$T = \begin{bmatrix} T_{11} & T_{12} & T_{13} \\ T_{21} & T_{22} & T_{23} \\ T_{31} & T_{32} & 1 \end{bmatrix} \tag{2.27}$$

The parameters of the matrix can be determined using RANSAC [14]. If we define the transformation matrix between two successive images as $\mathbf{T}_{n,n-1}$, the total transformation between the first and the nth frame can be defined as follows:

$$T_{n,1} = T_{n,n-1} T_{n-1,n-2}, \ldots, T_{2,1} \tag{2.28}$$

Using these transformations, each image can be mapped to a reference coordinate frame. To find the key frames we look at the ratio of the overlapping pixels between successive frames; if it is smaller than a threshold, we add the current frame to the list of key frames. In Fig. 2.10, key frames and the resulting panorama are shown for a sample video sequence. The original sequence has 260 frames, but in the panorama it can be represented with only four key frames when 50% overlap is assumed between frames.

As we can see from the figure, as we near the edges of the panorama, projective transform results in large warped images. We can use cylindrical projections to prevent the panorama from becoming too large. When the

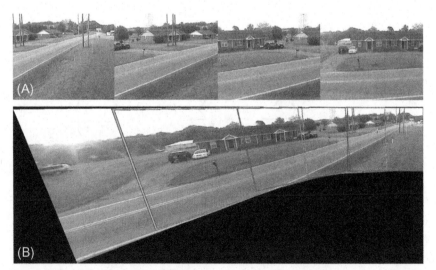

Figure 2.10 (A) Key frames and (B) resulting panorama from a sample video sequence. Key frames are marked with rectangles in the panorama. *(The video is from [15]).*

camera is only panning or tilting without rotations or zooming, the camera movement can be represented as translations in cylindrical coordinates [14]. For Cartesian image coordinates (x_c, y_c), their cylindrical projections, (x_s, y_s) can be found as follows:

$$x_s = f \arctan \left(\frac{x_c}{f} \right)$$
$$y_s = f \frac{y}{\sqrt{x_c^2 + y_c^2}}$$

(2.29)

where f denotes the focal length of the camera. In Fig. 2.11, the results of cylindrical projections on the same video sequence are displayed.

SURF method works best when the images have well-defined edges as in the above examples. However, we observed that it can fail to register images in videos recorded with wildfire surveillance cameras in less than ideal conditions as shown in Fig. 2.12, as we can see the images are blurry and the edges are not very distinctive. With these images SURF method fails to find enough inliers (matching feature locations), but we can use MI-based optimization to register the images.

After finding the key frames, the real-time processing needs to register each new image to a key frame and update the background. For the first new frame we search the whole key frame dataset, for the other frames we look for a subset of the key frames that are close to the previously selected

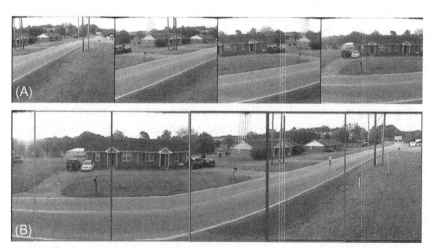

Figure 2.11 (A) Key frames and (B) resulting panorama in cylindrical coordinates from a sample video sequence. Key frames are marked with rectangles in the panorama. *(The video is from [15]).*

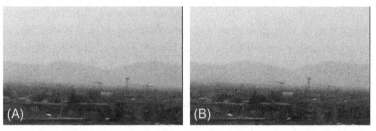

Figure 2.12 Wildfire surveillance images: (A) current frame, (B) next frame.

key frame. We observed that matching the current frame to the key frames is best accomplished using MI, instead of SURF features. We show an example of this for the image set in Fig. 2.13. The panorama scene provides 180° coverage with 1300 frames which is represented by 18 key frames with 75% overlap between them. Fig. 2.14 shows the frame index versus key frame index for this video sequence for both MI and SURF methods. We see that MI method shifts between the key frames without any distortions, while SURF method oscillates between neighboring frames. When we use the MI method, the reference key frame is the same for 60 frames on the average. This means that the locations of the wildfire region will be the same for this time interval. We can then extract spatiotemporal features from the subset of the video sequence that characterize the wildfire behavior.

2.8.2 Wildfire Detection Algorithm

The wildfire detection algorithm consists of the following main steps: background subtraction using registered images, color analysis, robust feature analysis, spatiotemporal feature extraction, and classification. We use an infinite impulse response (IIR) filter-based background subtraction method defined in [16]. We use a large update parameter to adapt to slow update periods caused by the continuous movement of the camera. After background subtraction, we perform color analysis of detected regions to determine candidate smoke regions. Wildfire smoke usually has a gray-to-white color that results from burning vegetation. We use thresholds in YUV color space to determine color content of regions. The color condition is defined as follows [17]:

$$M_C = Y > T_Y \& |U - 128| < T_U \& |V - 128| < T_V \qquad (2.30)$$

where Y, U, V denote separate channels of the color space, T_Y, T_U, and T_V are predetermined thresholds, and M_C is the color mask for the whole image.

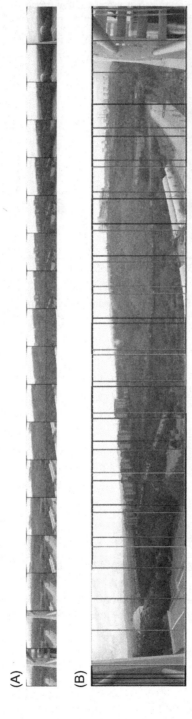

Figure 2.13 (A) Key frames and (B) resulting panorama in cylindrical coordinates from a sample video sequence. Key frames are marked with rectangles in the panorama.

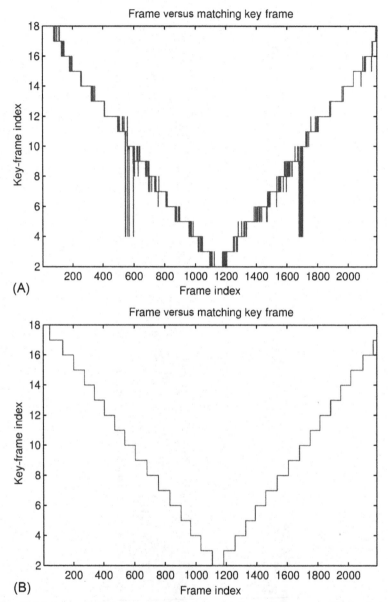

Figure 2.14 Frame index versus key frame index for real-time operation using the background panorama of Fig. 2.13b: (A) SURF method, (B) MI method.

Another observation about the smoke regions is that they are usually smoother than the surrounding background covered with trees and irregular terrain. We exploit this observation by masking the regions around the SURF features according to their scale values.

2.8.2.1 Feature Extraction

For each spatiotemporal block, if the ratio of the pixels satisfying the color condition is above a threshold, this block is further processed for feature extraction and classification. We use an LBPs-based feature extraction method. We propose two improvements to achieve real-time performance by reducing the computational cost of the method. We use random sampling to significantly reduce the computational cost of LBP method. We show that using random hyperplanes to reduce the dimension of feature vectors can decrease computational cost and preserve classification accuracy.

In data mining applications, hashing functions are used to reduce the dimensionality of the data and provide fast access to large databases. One of the dimension reduction methods used for hashing is the random hyperplane method used with inner product similarity [18]. Let us assume that x is a $Q \times 1$ vector representing the dynamic texture of video signal. Φ represents a random hyperplane with the same dimensions as x and its elements are obtained from a standard normal distribution. The hash function for the feature vector is obtained as $h\Phi = \text{sign}(\Phi Tx)$. When P different random hyperplanes are used, P-bit low-dimensional representation for the feature is obtained. In our application, we do not use the sign function and directly use the result of the inner product to find the reduced feature vectors.

LBPs are first introduced for texture classification [19]. In this method each pixel in the image is compared to its predefined number of neighbors. If the center pixel's value is larger than its neighbor, it is marked with 1, and marked with 0 otherwise. The binary values form the k-digit number where k is the number of neighbors. The histogram of all binary numbers corresponding to pixels form the LBP feature vector. The extension of the LBP method to image sequences is proposed in [20]. VLBP method uses three parallel planes in the time axis to form the feature vector. The binary number is obtained from the neighbors in all three planes. Therefore the dimension of the feature vector increases exponentially with the number of neighbors. LBP-TOP method decreases the dimension of the feature vector by considering three orthogonal planes around the center pixels and calculating the binary number separately for each plane. The final feature vector is obtained by concatenating the histograms corresponding to each orthogonal plane.

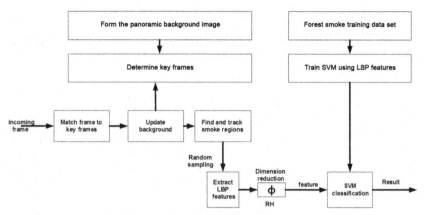

Figure 2.15 Overview of the proposed feature extraction method.

In our application we accumulate the detection results from a smoke region that is registered to the same key frame. The dimension of the block is $WB \times HB \times FB$. We generate a random grid of coordinates with G elements that fall within the volume corresponding to the spatiotemporal smoke region. We calculate $3 \times 2k$ dimensional LBP feature vectors for each random coordinate for user-selected k neighbors. We use standard normal distributed P random hyperplanes of size $1 \times (3 \times 2k)$ for dimensionality reduction. When we multiply the LBP feature vector with the random hyperplanes we get a feature vector of size $P \leq 3 \times 1$. The overview of the wildfire detection process is shown in Fig. 2.15.

The random sampling and dimension reduction steps can provide multiple orders of magnitude speedup in feature extraction and classification without decreasing the success rate. As an example for blocks of size $16 \times 16 \times 64$, the standard LBP requires 16384 LBP calculations. If we use only 1024 random samples we can get $16 \times$ theoretical speed up. We perform extensive experiments to validate the proposed methods. We use support vector machines (SVM) for classification [21].

2.8.3 Experimental Results

In the first part of the experiments, we present the classification results for the feature extraction process. We use training and test videos that are obtained from various wildfire surveillance towers and under different conditions. In the dataset we have 13 videos that contain actual smoke (positive videos) and 12 videos that contain smoke–colored moving regions (negative videos) that cause false alarms. We use one-fifth of the video sequences for training and the rest for testing. We define the methods compared in the experiments below:

- LBP4: Full LBP method with 4-neighborhood.
- LBP8: Full LBP method with 8-neighborhood.
- RS1000LBP4: 4-neighborhood LBP method calculated with randomly sampled 1000 coordinates.
- RS1000LBP8: 8-neighborhood LBP method calculated with randomly sampled 1000 coordinates.
- RH16RS1000LBP4: 4-neighborhood LBP method calculated with randomly sampled 1000 coordinates after dimension reduction using 16 random hyperplanes with a Gaussian vector of size 1×48.
- RH128RS1000LBP8: 4-neighborhood LBP method calculated with randomly sampled 1000 coordinates after dimension reduction using 128 random hyperplanes with a Gaussian vector of size 1×768.

Table 2.2 shows the classification results for the wildfire smoke dataset. In the training set we have 34,798 and 57,507 samples from positive and negative videos, respectively. In the table we show the results when we only use a fraction of the training set to see the generalization performance of the classifier. For each $16 \times 16 \times 64$ spatiotemporal block we only use randomly selected 1000 points for LBP calculations.

From the results we see that 128-dimensional feature vectors of RH128RS1000LBP8 perform very close to 768-dimensional feature vectors of RS1000LBP8. When one-eighth of the training set is used, the success rate in the test set is %96.68 for RH, which is quite satisfactory for this problem.

Table 2.2 Wildfire smoke recognition success rates (percentage)

Smoke dataset: c_1: 34798 c_2: 57507

Method	NS/128	NS/64	NS/32	NS/16	NS/8
RS1000LBP4	87.02	90.19	92.72	94.09	95.17
RS1000LBP8	87.50	89.67	91.13	94.15	97.01
RH24RS1000LBP4	84.92	87.85	89.02	90.08	91.11
RH128RS1000LBP8	88.29	91.54	94.08	95.66	96.68

In the ratio NS/a, ns denotes the total number of training samples and a is the ratio of the training set that is used. C_i denotes the number of samples for the ith class.

Table 2.3 Number of support vectors/total classification time (s) for smoke detection dataset

Smoke dataset: c_1: 34798 c_2: 57507

Method	NS/128	NS/64	NS/32	NS/16	NS/8
RS1000LBP4	181/ 1.73	332/ 3.24	576/5.57	1049/ 10.11	1916/ 17.87
RS1000LBP8	321/ 65.09	466/ 77.82	687/ 132.28	1023/ 170.59	1798/ 230.60
RP24RS1000LBP4	210/ 1.44	409/ 2.64	793/5.08	1507/9.52	2856/ 15.73
RP128RS1000LBP8	202/ 4.15	327/ 6.62	583/ 11.74	975/20.73	1698/ 38.12

Another important criteria for SVM classification is the number of support vectors of the model. Table 2.3 shows the number of support vectors and total classification time (seconds) for the dataset configuration in Table 2.2. $RH_{128}RS_{1000}LBP_8$ method usually has lower number of support vectors and its classification time is significantly less than $RS_{1000}LBP_8$ method.

In the next part of the experiments we demonstrate sample detection results from videos recorded with continuously panning cameras. Fig. 2.16 shows detection results for the video sequence in Fig. 2.13.

In Fig. 2.17 results from a 360° coverage panorama is shown. The panorama uses 113 key frames to represent a full scan of the camera consisting of 9000 frames. We see that the system detects the wildfire smoke even when the image quality is poor with the help of the MI method.

2.8.4 Conclusion

In conclusion, we developed a real-time wildfire detection algorithm to reduce the scanning period of conventional stop-and-detect methods by using continuously moving cameras. We investigated the performance of SURF features in low-quality images recorded with wildfire surveillance cameras. We showed that MI-based methods can provide robustness against low-quality images during the registration process. We proposed a wildfire detection method that can exploit robust features to characterize smoke behavior. Experimental results for feature extraction and real-time tests prove the performance of the proposed algorithm.

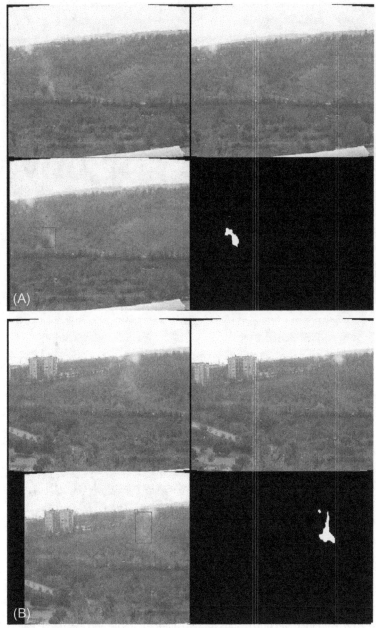

Figure 2.16 Wildfire detection results for two different frame and key frame pairs using the video sequence from Fig. 2.13. Top-left image is the current frame, top-right image is the corresponding key frame, bottom-left image is the registered current image, bottom-right image is the candidate smoke region.

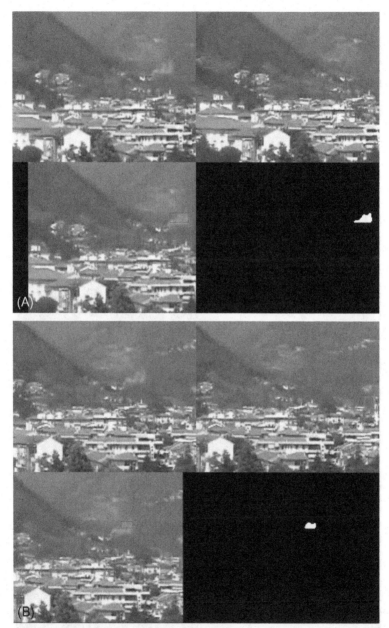

Figure 2.17 Wildfire detection results for two different frame and key frame pairs using the 360° coverage video sequence. Top-left image is the current frame, top-right image is the corresponding key frame, bottom-left image is the registered current image, bottom-right image is the candidate smoke region.

REFERENCES

[1] D. Lowe, Distinctive image features from scale-invariant keypoints, Int. J. Comput. Vis. 60 (2) (2004) 91–110. [Online]. Available: http://dx.doi.org/10.1023/B% 3AVISI.0000029664.99615.94.

[2] W.M.W. III, P.A. Viola, H. Atsumi, Multi-modal volume registration by maximization of mutual information, Med. Image Anal. 1 (1) (1996) 35–51.

[3] E. Monari, T. Pollok, A real-time image-to-panorama registration approach for background subtraction using pan-tilt-cameras, in: Advanced Video and Signal-Based Surveillance (AVSS), 2011 8th IEEE International Conference on, Aug 2011, 2011, pp. 237–242.

[4] L. Zeng, S. Zhang, J. Zhang, Y. Zhang, Dynamic image mosaic via sift and dynamic programming, Mach. Vis. Appl. 25 (5) (2014) 1271–1282. [Online]. Available:http:// dx.doi.org/10.1007/s00138-013-0551-8.

[5] M. Uyttendaele, A. Eden, R. Szeliski, Eliminating ghosting and exposure artifacts in image mosaics, in: IEEE Computer Society Conference on Computer Vision and Pattern Recognition (CVPR), vol. II, IEEE Computer Society, Kauai, Hawaii, 2001, pp. 509–516. [Online]. Available: http://research.microsoft.com/apps/pubs/ default.aspx?id=75702.

[6] A. Bevilacqua, P. Azzari, High-quality real time motion detection using PTZ cameras, in: IEEE International Conference on Video and Signal Based Surveillance (AVSS), 2006p. 23.

[7] K. Pulli, M. Tico, Y. Xiong, Mobile panoramic imaging system, in: IEEE Computer Society Conference on Computer Vision and Pattern Recognition Workshops (CVPRW), 2010, pp. 108–115.

[8] M. Fadaeieslam, M. Fathy, M. Soryani, Key frames selection into panoramic mosaics, in: International Conference on Information, Communications and Signal Processing (ICICS), 2009, pp. 1–5.

[9] C. Arth, M. Klopschitz, G. Reitmayr, D. Schmalstieg, Real-time self-localization from panoramic images on mobile devices, in: IEEE International Symposium on Mixed and Augmented Reality (ISMAR), 2011, pp. 37–46.

[10] X. Mei, M. Ramachandran, S. Zhou, Video background retrieval using mosaic images, in: IEEE International Conference on Acoustics, Speech, and Signal Processing, 2005. Proceedings (ICASSP), vol. 2, 2005, pp. 441–444.

[11] P. Azzari, L. Di Stefano, A. Bevilacqua, An effective real-time mosaicing algorithm apt to detect motion through background subtraction using a PTZ camera, in: IEEE Conference on Advanced Video and Signal Based Surveillance (AVSS), 2005, pp. 511–516.

[12] D. Wagner, A. Mulloni, T. Langlotz, D. Schmalstieg, Real-time panoramic mapping and tracking on mobile phones, in: Virtual Reality Conference (VR), 2010 IEEE, 2010, pp. 211–218.

[13] H. Bay, A. Ess, T. Tuytelaars, L.V. Gool, Speeded-up robust features (surf), Comput. Vis. Image Underst. 110 (3) (2008) 346–359. similarity Matching in Computer Vision and Multimedia. [Online]. Available: http://www.sciencedirect.com/science/arti cle/pii/S1077314207001555.

[14] R. Szeliski, Image Alignment and Stitching: A Tutorial, Microsoft Research, Tech. Rep. MSR-TR-2004-92, October 2004. [Online]. Available: http://research. microsoft.com/apps/pubs/default.aspx?id=70092.

[15] N. Goyette, P. Jodoin, F. Porikli, J. Konrad, P. Ishwar, Changedetection.net: a new change detection benchmark dataset, in: IEEE Computer Society Conference on Computer Vision and Pattern Recognition Workshops (CVPRW), 2012, pp. 1–8.

[16] R. Collins, A. Lipton, T. Kanade, H. Fujiyoshi, D. Duggins, Y. Tsin, D. Tolliver, N. Enomoto, O. Hasegawa, A System for Video Surveillance and Monitoring, Robotics Institute, Pittsburgh, PA, Tech. Rep. CMU-RI-TR-00-12, May 2000.

[17] O. Gunay, B.U. Treyin, K. Kose, A.E. Cetin, Entropy-functional-based online adaptive decision fusion framework with application to wildfire detection in video, IEEE Trans. Image Process. 21 (5) (2012) 2853–2865.

[18] B. Kulis, K. Grauman, Kernelized locality-sensitive hashing for scalable image search, in: IEEE International Conference on Computer Vision (ICCV), 2009, pp. 2130–2137.

[19] T. Ojala, M. Pietikainen, D. Harwood, Performance evaluation of texture measures with classification based on kullback discrimination of distributions, in: IAPR International Conference on Pattern Recognition (ICPR), vol. 1, 1994, pp. 582–585.

[20] G. Zhao, M. Pietikainen, Dynamic texture recognition using local binary patterns with an application to facial expressions, IEEE Trans. Pattern Anal. Mach. Intell. 29 (6) (June 2007) 915–928.

[21] C.-C. Chang, C.-J. Lin, LIBSVM: a library for support vector machines, 2001. Software available at http://www.csie.ntu.edu.tw/~cjlin/libsvm.

[22] O. Günay, Video processing algorithms for wildfire surveillance, PhD. Thesis, Bilkent University, Electrical and Electronics Engineering, 2015.

CHAPTER 3

Infrared Sensor-Based Flame Detection

Contents

Conventional point smoke and fire detectors typically detect the presence of certain particles generated by smoke and fire by ionization or photometry. An important weakness of point detectors is that the smoke has to reach the sensor. This may take a significant amount of time to issue an alarm and therefore it is not possible to use them in open spaces or large rooms. The main advantage of differential pyroelectric infrared (PIR)-based sensor system for fire detection over the conventional smoke detectors is the ability to monitor large rooms and spaces because they analyze the infrared light reflected from hot objects or fire flames to reach a decision.

An uncontrolled fire in its early stage exhibits a transition to chaos due to the fact that the combustion process consists of nonlinear instabilities which result in transition to chaotic behavior via intermittency [1–5]. Consequently, turbulent flames can be characterized as a chaotic wide band frequency activity. Therefore, it is not possible to observe a single flickering frequency in the light spectrum due to an uncontrolled fire. In fact, we obtained a time series from the sampled read-out signal strength values of a PIR sensor with flickering flames in its viewing range (cf. Fig. 3.3). It is clear from Fig. 3.3 that there is no single flickering frequency and that flame flicker behavior is a wide-band activity covering 1-13 Hz. It is also reported in the literature that turbulent flames of an uncontrolled fire flicker with a frequency of around 10 Hz [6,7]. Actually, instantaneous flame flicker frequency is not constant, rather it varies in time. Recently developed

Methods and Techniques for Fire Detection
http://dx.doi.org/10.1016/B978-0-12-802399-0.00003-X

video-based fire detection schemes also take advantage of this fact by detecting random high-frequency behavior in flame colored moving pixels [8–10]. Therefore, a Markov model-based modeling of flame flicker process produces a more robust performance compared to frequency domain-based methods. Markov models are extensively used in speech recognition systems and in computer vision applications [11–14].

In [15] and [16], several experiments on the relationship between burner size and flame flicker frequency are presented. Recent research on pyro-IR based combustion monitoring includes [17] in which monitoring system using an array of PIR detectors is realized.

A regular camera or typical IR flame sensors have a fire detection range of 30 m. The detection range of an ordinary low-cost PIR sensor-based system is 10 m but this is enough to cover most rooms with high ceilings. Therefore, PIR-based systems provide a cost-effective solution to the fire detection problem in relatively large rooms as the unit cost of a camera-based system or a regular IR sensor-based system is in the order of one thousand dollars.

In the proposed approach, wavelet domain signal processing methods are used for feature extraction from sensor signals. This provides robustness against sensor signal drift due to temperature variations in the observed area. Notice that differential PIR sensors are sensitive only to the changes in the intensity of the IR radiation within the viewing range, rather than the absolute infrared radiation. In a very hot room the differential PIR sensor does not measure the temperature of the room; it only produces a constant output value which is not related to the temperature value. Regular temperature changes in a room are slow variations compared to the moving objects and flames. Since wavelet signals are high-pass and band-pass signals, they do not get affected by slow variations in sensor signal.

There are two different classes of events defined in this approach. The first class represents fire events whereas the second class represents non-fire events. Each class of events is modeled by a different Markov model. The main application of PIR sensors is hot body motion detection. Therefore, we include regular human motion events like walking or running in the non-fire event class.

In Section 3.1, we present the operating principles of PIR sensors and how we modified the PIR circuit for flame detection. In Section 3.2, the wavelet domain signal processing and the Markov-based modeling of the flames and human motion are described. In Section 3.3, comparative experimental results with other sensing modalities are presented.

3.1 OPERATING PRINCIPLES OF A PIR SENSOR SYSTEM AND DATA ACQUISITION

The main motivation of using a PIR sensor is that it can reliably detect the presence of moving bodies from other objects. Basically, it detects the difference in infrared radiation between the two "segments" in its viewing range. Sensing normal variations in temperature and also disturbances in airflow are avoided by the elements connected in pairs. When these elements are subject to the same infrared radiation level, they generate a zero-output signal by canceling each other out [18]. Therefore, a PIR sensor can reject false detections accurately. The block diagram of a typical differential PIR sensor is shown in Fig. 3.1. A single sensor system requires additional expensive IR filters to distinguish ordinary hot bodies from CO and CO_2 emissions. In this chapter, we show that it is possible to distinguish the flames from other hot bodies by analyzing the motion information captured by the differential PIR system.

Commercially available PIR motion-detector readout circuits produce binary outputs. However, it is possible to capture a continuous time analog signal indicating the strength of the received signal in time. The circuit diagram of a typical PIR motion-detector is shown in Fig. 3.2. It is possible to capture an analog signal from this circuit.

The circuit consists of four operational amplifiers (op amps), IC1A, IC1B, IC1C, and IC1D. IC1A and B constitute a two-stage amplifier

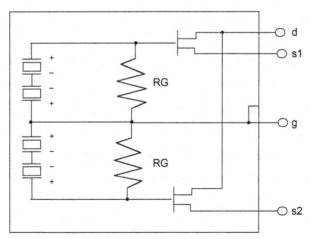

Figure 3.1 The model of the internal structure of a PIR sensor.

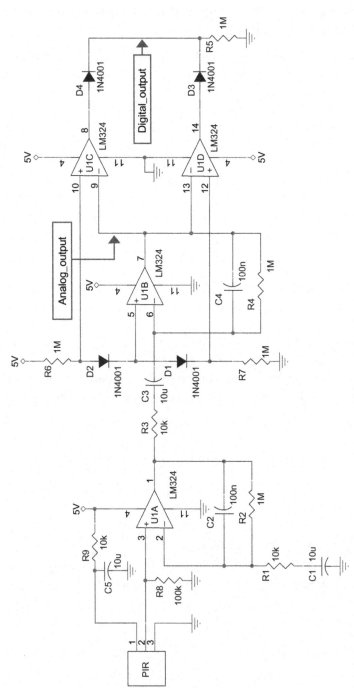

Figure 3.2 The circuit diagram for capturing an analog signal output from a PIR sensor.

circuit, whereas IC1C and D couple behaves as a comparator. The very-low amplitude raw output at the second pin of the PIR sensor is amplified through the two-stage amplifier circuit. The amplified signal at the output of IC1B is fed into the comparator structure which outputs a binary signal, either 0 or 5 V. Instead of using binary output in the original version of the PIR sensor readout circuit, we directly capture the analog output signal at the output of the second op amp, IC1B and transfer it to a computer or a digital signal processor for further processing. The goal is to distinguish the flame signal from other signals due to ordinary moving bodies.

In uncontrolled fires, flames flicker. Following the discussion in Section 3.1 regarding the turbulent wide band activity of flame flicker process, the analog signal is sampled with a sampling frequency of $f_s = 50$ Hz because the highest flame flicker frequency is 13 Hz and $f_s = 50$ Hz and is well above the Nyquist rate, 2×13 Hz [7]. In Fig. 3.3, a frequency distribution plot corresponding to a flickering flame of an uncontrolled fire is shown. It is clear that the sampling frequency of 50 Hz is sufficient. Typical sampled signal for no activity case using 8 bit quantization is shown in Fig. 3.4. Other typical received signals from a moving person and flickering fire are presented in Figs. 3.5 and 3.6, respectively.

The strength of the received signal from a differential PIR sensor increases when there is motion due to a hot body within its viewing range. In fact, this is due to the fact that pyroelectric sensors give an electric response to a rate of change of temperature rather than temperature itself. On the other hand, the motion may be due to human motion taking place in front of the sensors or flickering flame. In this chapter, the differential PIR sensor data is used to distinguish the flame flicker from the motion of a human being, such as running or walking. Typically the PIR signal

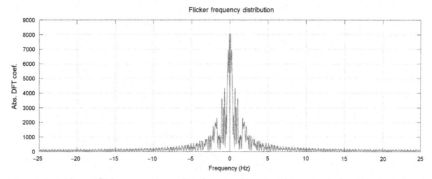

Figure 3.3 Flame flicker spectrum distribution. PIR signal is sampled with 50 Hz.

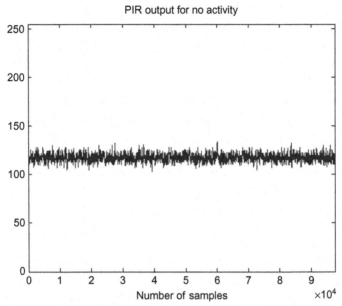

Figure 3.4 A typical PIR sensor output sampled at 50 Hz with 8 bit quantization when there is no activity within its viewing range.

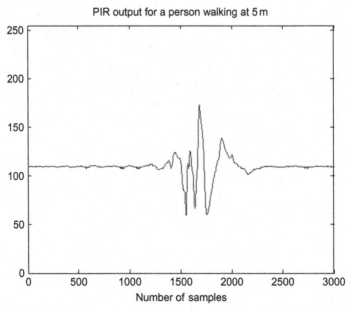

Figure 3.5 PIR sensor output signal recorded at a distance of 5 m for a walking person.

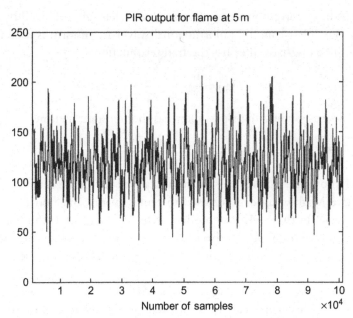

Figure 3.6 PIR sensor output signal recorded at a distance of 5 m for a flame of an uncontrolled fire.

frequency of oscillation for a flickering flame is higher than that of PIR signals caused by a moving hot body. In order to keep the computational cost of the detection mechanism low, we decided to use Lagrange filters for obtaining the wavelet transform coefficients as features instead of using a direct frequency approach, such as the Fast Fourier Transform (FFT)-based methods.

3.2 SENSOR DATA PROCESSING AND MARKOV MODELS

Two different Markov models corresponding to flames and other motion are trained using the wavelet transforms of PIR recordings. Training of Markov models are carried out using various fire and motion recordings. During testing, the sensor signal is fed to both Markov models and the model producing the highest probability determines the class of the signal.

There is a bias in the PIR sensor output signal which changes according to the room temperature. Wavelet transform of the PIR signal removes this bias. Let $x[n]$ be a sampled version of the signal coming out of a PIR sensor. Wavelet coefficients obtained after a single-stage sub-band decomposition, $w[k]$, corresponding to (12.5 Hz, 25 Hz) frequency band information of the original sensor output signal $x[n]$ are evaluated with an integer arithmetic high-pass filter corresponding to Lagrange wavelets [19] followed by deci-mation. The filter bank of a biorthogonal wavelet transform is used in the analysis. The low-pass filter has the transfer function

$$H_l(z) = \frac{1}{2} + \frac{1}{4}\left(z^{-1} + z^1\right) \qquad (3.1)$$

and the corresponding high-pass filter has the transfer function

$$H_h(z) = \frac{1}{2} - \frac{1}{4}\left(z^{-1} + z^1\right) \qquad (3.2)$$

A Markov model-based classification is carried out for fire detection. Two three-state Markov models are used to represent fire and non-fire events (cf. Fig. 3.7). In these Markov models, state $S1$ corresponds to no activity within the viewing range of the PIR sensor. The system remains in state $S1$ as long as there is not any significant activity, which means that the absolute value of the current wavelet coefficient at index number k, $|w[k]|$, is below a nonnegative threshold T, where T is initialized based on the background noise level. This value can be estimated by a genetic algorithm-based approach, as in [20]. The second state, $S2$, which corresponds to an increase, or "rise" in consecutive wavelet coefficient values, is attained when

$$w[k] - w[k-1] > T \qquad (3.3)$$

is satisfied. Similarly, the third state, $S3$, which corresponds to a decrease, or "fall" in consecutive wavelet coefficient values, is attained when

$$w[k] - w[k-1] < T \qquad (3.4)$$

is satisfied.

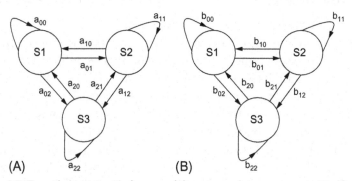

Figure 3.7 Two three-state Markov models are used to represent (A) "fire" and (B) "non-fire" classes, respectively.

The first step of the Markov-based analysis consists of dividing the wavelet coefficient sequences in windows of 25 samples. For each window, a corresponding state transition sequence is determined. An example state transition sequence of size 5 may look like:

$$C = \{S2, S1, S3, S2, S1\} \tag{3.5}$$

Since the wavelet signal captures the high frequency information in the signal, we expect that there will be more transitions occurring between states when monitoring fire compared to human motion.

The threshold T in the wavelet domain determines the state transition probabilities, given a signal. In the training step, given T, ground-truth fire and non-fire wavelet training sequences, the task is to estimate the transition probabilities for each class. Let a_{ij} denote the transition probabilities for the "fire" class and b_{ij} denote the transition probabilities for the "non-fire" class.

The decision about the class affiliation of a state transition sequence C of size L is made by calculating the two joint probabilities $P_a(C)$ and $P_b(C)$ corresponding to fire and non-fire classes, respectively:

$$P_a(C) = \prod_i p_a(C_{i+1}|C_i) = \prod_i a_{C_i, C_{i+1}}, \tag{3.6}$$

and

$$P_b(C) = \prod_i p_b(C_{i+1}|C_i) = \prod_i b_{C_i, C_{i+1}} \tag{3.7}$$

where $p_a(C_{i+1}|C_i) = a_{C_i, C_{i+1}}$, and $p_b(C_{i+1}|C_i) = b_{C_i, C_{i+1}}$, and $i = 1,...,L$.

In case of $P_a(C) > P_b(C)$, the class affiliation of state transition sequence C will be declared as "fire," otherwise it is declared as "non-fire."

For the training of the Markov models, the state transition probabilities for human motion and flame are estimated from 250 consecutive wavelet coefficients covering a time frame of 10 s.

During the classification phase, a state history signal consisting of 50 consecutive wavelet coefficients are computed from the received sensor signal. This state sequence is fed to fire and non-fire Markov models for each window. The model yielding the highest probability is determined as the result of the analysis of PIR sensor data.

For flame sequences, the transition probabilities a's should be high and close to each other due to random nature of uncontrolled fire. On the other hand, transition probabilities should be small in constant temperature moving bodies like a walking person because there is no change or little change in sensor signal values. Hence, we expect a higher probability for b_{00} than any other b value in the non-fire model which corresponds to higher probability of being in $S1$. The states $S2$ and $S3$ aim at tracking the rising and falling trends of the sensor signal in wavelet domain, respectively. Therefore, we expect frequent transitions between these states for uncontrolled fire.

3.3 EXPERIMENTAL RESULTS

The analog output signal is sampled with a sampling frequency of 50 Hz and quantized at 8 bits. Real-time analysis and classification methods are implemented with C++ running on a PC. Digitized output signal is fed to the PC via RS-232 serial port. It is also possible to process this signal using a Field Programmable Gate Array (FPGA) or a digital signal processor.

In our experiments, we recorded fire and non-fire sequences at a distance of 5 m to the sensor. For fire sequences, we burned paper and alcohol, and recorded the output signals. For the non-fire sequences, we recorded walking and running person sequences. The person within the viewing range of the PIR sensor walked or ran in a straight line which was tangent to the circle with a radius of 5 m and the sensor being at the center.

The training set consists of 90 fire and 90 non-fire recordings with durations varying between 3 and 4 s. The test set for fire class is 220 and that of non-fire set is 593. Our method successfully detected fire for 217 of the sequences in the fire test set. It did not trigger fire alarm for any of the sequences in the non-fire test set. This is presented in Table 3.1.

The false negative alarms, 3 out of 220 fire test sequences, were issued for the recordings where a man was also within the viewing range of the sensor along with a fire inside a wastebasket. The test setting for which false alarms are issued is shown in Fig. 3.8. The system was tested live at a trade show for three days in Valladolid, Spain in November 2010. This was a FIRESENSE project activity [21]. The flame detector did not produce any false alarms and it detected flames in 30 cm almost instantaneously.

Table 3.1 Results with 220 fire, 593 non-fire test sequences

	Number of sequences	Number of false alarms	Number of alarms
Fire test sequences	220	3	217
Non-fire test sequences	593	0	0

The system triggers an alarm when fire is detected within the viewing range of the PIR sensor.

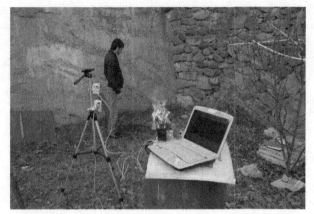

Figure 3.8 The PIR sensor is encircled. The fire is close to die out completely. A man is also within the viewing range of the sensor.

We also tested and compared several commercial smoke and fire sensors. The first test area was a 4- by 4-meter small room with a ceiling height of 2.5 m. The test fire was burnt in a 40×25 cm barbecue chamber. The test fire was also recorded by an IPX DDK-1500 video camera from a distance of 2.5 m. The PIR flame detection sensor system is based on the PARADOX motion detector.

The following sensors were used: Flamingo FA11 photo electric smoke sensor, CATA–CT9451 smoke alarm sensor, and CODE DN-23 optical smoke detector. All of the sensors were placed directly above the fire pan. Under the given test conditions, response times for the sensors are given in Table 3.2. The differential PIR sensor response is better than two smoke detectors even for such small rooms. It is obviously slower than video flame and smoke detectors, but they are expensive systems requiring computer processing.

Table 3.2 Response times of different sensors

	Response time
Paradox PIR flame sensor	1 min 48 s
Flamingo FA11 photo electric smoke sensor	1 min 17 s
CATA-CT9451 smoke alarm sensor	9 min 36 s
CODEDN-23 optical smoke detector	11 min 32 s
IPXDDK-1500 video camera (as smoke detector)	Less than 10 s
IPXDDK-1500 video camera (as flame detector)	Less than 5 s

Table 3.3 Comparison of the responses of Paradox PIR flame sensor and Flamingo FA11 photo electric smoke sensor to the flame in a barbecue, at 4-6 m distance, in a 10 m × 9 m × 3.5 m room

Fire area	Fire height	Distance	Alarm time	
			Paradox PIR flame sensor	Flamingo FA11 photo electric smoke sensor
0.04532 m^2	30 cm	4 m	25 s	No alarm
0.06265 m^2	40 cm	4 m	19 s	No alarm
0.08814 m^2	65 cm	4 m	8 s	No alarm
0.09823 m^2	75 cm	4 m	7 s	No alarm
0.12150 m^2	80 cm	4 m	5 s	No alarm
0.08679 m^2	90 cm	6 m	21 s	No alarm

In the second case, the differential PIR sensor system was tested in a large 10- by 12-meter room with a ceiling of 5 m. The distance between the 30 cm diameter pan and the PIR sensor was 9 m. The PIR sensor responded the flames in 35 s after they became visible. We burned cardboard inside the flames. The response time was less than 2 min after ignition. In this case, none of the smoke sensors could issue an alarm within 10 min.

Finally, we tested the Paradox PIR flame sensor and Flamingo FA11 Photo Electric Smoke Sensor in a 10- by 9-meter room with a ceiling of 3.5 m. The distance between the sensors and the flame in a barbecue of 40 cm diameter was 4-6 m. The Flamingo FA11 photo electric smoke sensor could not produce an alarm within 30 min, but the differential PIR sensor responded in a very short time. The results are presented in Table 3.3.

REFERENCES

[1] F. Erden, B. Ugur Toreyin, E. Birey Soyer, I. Inac, O. Gunay, K. Kose, A. Enis Cetin, Wavelet based flickering flame detector using differential PIR sensors, Fire Saf. J. 0379-711253 (2012) 13–18. http://dx.doi.org/10.1016/j.firesaf.2012.06.006.
[2] C.K. Law, Combustion Physics, Cambridge University Press, New York, NY, 2006. http://www.amazon.com/Combustion-Physics-Chung-K-Law/dp/0521870526/ ref=mt_hardcover?_encoding=UTF8&me=.
[3] V. Gubernov, A. Kolobov, A. Polezhaev, H. Sidhu, G. Mercer, Period doubling and chaotic transient in a model of chain-branching combustion wave propagation, Proc. R. Soc. Lond. A 466 (2121) (2010) 2747–2769.
[4] M. Wendeker, J. Czarnigowski, G. Litak, K. Szabelski, Chaotic combustion in spark ignition engines, Chaos, Solitons Fractals 18 (2004) 805–808.
[5] P. Manneville, Instabilities, Chaos and Turbulence, Imperial College Press, London, 2004.

[6] S.A. Fastcom Technology, Method and Device for Detecting Fires Based on Image Analysis, 2002. PCT Pubn. No. WO02/069292, CH-1006, Lausanne, Switzerland.

[7] B.W. Albers, A.K. Agrawal, Schlieren analysis of an oscillating gas-jet diffusion, Combust. Flame 119 (1999) 84–94.

[8] W. Phillips III, M. Shah, N.V. Lobo, Flame recognition in video, Pattern Recogn. Lett. 23 (2002) 319–327.

[9] T. Chen, P. Wu, Y. Chiou, An early fire-detection method based on image processing, in: Proceedings of the International Conference on Image Processing (ICIP), 2004, pp. 1707–1710.

[10] B.U. Toreyin, Y. Dedeoglu, U. Gudukbay, A.E. Cetin, Computer vision based system for real-time fire and flame detection, Pattern Recogn. Lett. 27 (2006) 49–58.

[11] B.U. Toreyin, Y. Dedeoglu, A.E. Cetin, HMM based falling person detection using both audio and video, in: Proceedings of IEEE International Workshop on Human-Computer Interaction, Beijing, China, 2005, pp. 211–220.

[12] F. Jabloun, A.E. Cetin, The Teager energy based feature parameters for robust speech recognition in car noise, in: Proceedings of IEEE International Conf. on Acoustics, Speech, and Signal Processing (ICASSP'99), 1999, pp. 273–276.

[13] H. Bunke, T. Caelli, HMMs Applications in Computer Vision, World Scientific, 2001. http://www.amazon.com/Hidden-markov-models-applications-Intelligence/dp/ 9810245645.

[14] L.R. Rabiner, B.H. Juang, Fundamentals of Speech Recognition, Prentice-Hall, New Jersey, 1993.

[15] M. Thuillard, A new flame detector using the latest research on flames and fuzzy-wavelet algorithms, Fire Saf. J. 37 (2002) 371–380.

[16] M. Thuillard, Wavelets in soft computing, World Scientific Publishing, Singapore, 2001. https://books.google.com.tr/books?id=9fheTNfmdBkC&printsec=frontcover &source=gbs_ge_summary_r&cad=0#v=onepage&q&f=false.

[17] F.C. Carter, N. Cross, Combustion monitoring using infrared array-based detectors, Meas. Sci. Technol. 14 (2003) 1117–1122.

[18] S. Colliard-Piraud, "Signal conditioning for pyroelectric passive infrared (PIR) sensors," STMicroelectronics, AN4368 Application Note, Nov. 2013.

[19] C.W. Kim, R. Ansari, A.E. Cetin, A class of linear-phase regular biorthogonal wavelets, in: Proceedings of IEEE International Conf. on Acoustics, Speech, and Signal Processing (ICASSP'92), 1992, pp. 673–676.

[20] B.U. Toreyin, E.B. Soyer, O. Urfalioglu, A.E. Cetin, Flame detection system based on wavelet analysis of PIR sensor signals with an HMM decision mechanism, in: Proceedings of the EURASIP 16th European Signal Processing Conference (EUSIPCO 2008), 2008.

[21] O. Gunay, K. Tasdemir, B. Ugur Toreyin, A. Enis Cetin, Video based wild fire detection at night, Fire Saf. J. 44 (6) (2009) 860–868.

[22] B.U. Toreyin, E.B. Soyer, O. Urfalioglu, A.E. Cetin, Flame detection using PIR sensors, in: IEEE 16th Signal Processing, Communication and Applications Conference, SIU 2008, 2008.

[23] FIRESENSE, Fire detection and management through a multi-sensor network for the protection of cultural heritage areas from the risk of fire and extreme weather conditions, FP7-ENV-2009-1244088-FIRESENSE, http://www.firesense.eu, 2009.

[24] S. Verstockt, Multi-modal Video Analysis for Early Fire Detection, Ph.D. thesis, Ghent University, 2011.

CHAPTER 4

Multisensor Fire Analysis

Contents

4.1 INTRODUCTION

Until today, most of the fire alarms have had a very limited functionality. They generate an alarm when a specific threshold is reached and that's it. No specific information about the fire circumstances is given. However, in order to be able to help the fire crew in their decision-making process, it is important to know the evolution of the smoke and flames and to try to be faster than the fire. As such, besides timely and accurate detection, analysis, and forecasting is very important. Although, this is not an easy task, the experiments in this chapter show that, contrary to traditional detectors, video processing techniques can not only improve and accelerate the detection but also provide the analysis and the forecast of the fire. By running intelligent analysis techniques on the images of a video camera, valuable fire characteristics (eg, the flame size, smoke layer height, and the fire location) can be detected at the early stage of the fire and much more information concerning the fire spreading can be given. This gives the opportunity to generate different levels of alarms and to forward a detailed description of the fire event, together with the recorded video data, to the appropriate authorities (eg, operators and fire fighters).

A study of the literature revealed that the amount of research in this direction is limited. Even today, most fire alarm systems only detect the

Methods and Techniques for Fire Detection
http://dx.doi.org/10.1016/B978-0-12-802399-0.00004-1

presence of fire and are not able to model fire evolution. Even though the majority of these systems consist of several sensors monitoring the same scene, the analysis is usually carried out separately on each of the sensor's data streams. In order to perform more accurate detection and localization of smoke and flames, and to detect valuable fire characteristics at the early stage of the fire, we combine the detection results of each of these single-view cameras/sensors and analyze them together into a multisensor/multiview fire analysis set-up. The main goal of the proposed set-up is to provide a more valuable video fire analysis tool than the existing state-of-the-art (SOTA) work, where results are still limited and interpretation of the provided information is not straightforward.

The central research question of this chapter is: "Can we develop a framework to timely and accurately analyze the fire and can we use the extracted fire characteristics for video driven fire forecasting?" The first part of this chapter (Section 4.2) focuses on the SOTA methods and tools for video fire analysis and discusses their advantages and limitations. The results of these first approaches are still limited and interpretation of the provided information is not straightforward. As such, the main goal of our work is to provide a more valuable video fire analysis tool. The second part of this chapter (Section 4.3) presents our discrete wavelet transform (DWT) energy-based video smoke analysis and multimodal video flame spread measurement techniques. Subsequently, Section 4.4 discusses a multisensor extension to these video-based techniques. Since we have multiple cameras/sensors monitoring the scene from different viewpoints, problems that arise in one sensor can (most probably) be compensated by the others. This is also confirmed by several large-scale real-world fire experiments. Finally, we conclude this chapter in Section 4.5 and point out directions for future work.

4.2 STATE-OF-THE-ART IN VIDEO FIRE ANALYSIS

Only recently, a few approaches have been proposed in the literature that are capable of providing additional information on the fire circumstances, such as size and location. Yasmin [1] proposes a dynamic programming (DP) matching algorithm, which analyzes the set of contour pixels of subblocked binarized images from consecutive frames. For each of the contour pixels, the DP matching generates a displacement vector. These vectors are further analyzed by histogram analysis to obtain the orientation with the highest number of displacement vectors (ie, the global direction of the smoke). Despite the fact that this single-view approach offers some interesting insights, the output is very limited for further analysis, since it is restricted to four directions in two-dimensional (2D). Furthermore, it seems impossible to perform valuable fire analysis with one single camera, since a lot of crucial information can be missed. For example, when the propagation of the flames and/or smoke is not well aligned with the camera view, analysis of growing size and propagation becomes very complicated.

The system of Martinez-de Dios et al. [2] analyzes visual and IR movies of a propagating fire front in order to supply the time evolutions of the fire front shape and position, flame inclination angle, height and base width. As secondary outputs, their system also provides the fire front rate of spread (RoS) and a 3D graphical model of the fire front that can be rendered from any virtual view. The experimental setup of the system is illustrated in Fig. 4.1. The 3D model of the instantaneous fire front is constructed in real-time, based on measures of the fire front base (rear and leading edges position), and flame height and inclination angle. This graphical representation can be rendered from any point of view, simulating the image obtained by a virtual camera. Subjective evaluation of the 3D fire model viewed by Camera 3 (Fig. 4.1D) and the true image of Camera 3 (Fig. 4.1E) shows that their system achieves good performance. Although the system is directly aimed at, and is only demonstrated in laboratory experiments on a flat burn table, the authors indicate that it can also be extended to field applications [3,4]. However, as both the laboratory and the field tests require a frontal camera view (the camera axis is perpendicular to the fire front) and a lateral camera view (the camera axis is parallel to the fire front), questions do also arise about the system's real-world applicability. Furthermore, in order to estimate certain fire characteristics, such as the leading edge of the fire front, an observer must supply additional information about the fire "circumstances" (eg, the type of ignition) which further limits it suitability for fire analysis in real-world environments.

Similar lab experiments to those of Martinez-de Dios et al. are also discussed in [5]. In this work, Pastor et al. present a method for the fast and accurate calculation of the RoS by processing single-view infrared images. In order to calculate the RoS ($\sim$ flame front's position as a function of time) the correspondence between the coordinate system of the image (expressed in pixels) and the real coordinate system (expressed in meters) is needed. They propose to estimate this correspondence (ie, the homography matrix) using the direct linear transformation (DLT) algorithm. The same technique is used by Verstockt et al. in their video fire analysis framework proposed in [6]. A drawback of the system of Pastor et al. from our point of view is that it is based on an application for linear frame fronts that are generated on flat surfaces with known dimensions. Although technical guidelines are given for the extrapolation of their method to experimental scenarios on a larger

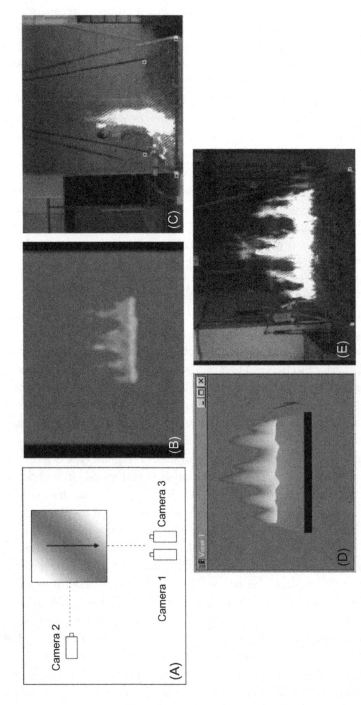

Figure 4.1 Video fire analysis system by Martinez-de Dios et al. [2]. Test with linear fire front, 30 s after ignition: (A) camera configuration; (B) image of Camera 1 (infrared, frontal); (C) image of Camera 2 (visual, lateral); (D) 3D fire model based on the images of Cameras 1 and 2, viewed by Camera 3 (virtual image); and (E) true image of Camera 3 (visual, frontal).

scale, they discuss themselves some problems/bottlenecks related to the system's applicability in a real-world environment. Furthermore, the assumption of a frontal view is again seen as a limitation.

Far more interesting than the prior approaches is the stereo vision work of Akhloufi and Rossi [7–9]. This approach, which is illustrated in Fig. 4.2, uses two stereo-vision cameras to track the fire spread in 3D space. First, a color-based segmentation is used to extract the fire regions from both cameras. These regions are then further analyzed by feature point detection and matching between the two camera images. Feature points (also called interest points or keypoints in literature) are locations in the image where the signal changes two-dimensionally, such as corners and line intersections, as well as locations where the texture varies significantly [10]. Based on the feature point matching, 3D fire points are computed using stereo correspondence. Finally, a 3D ellipsoid is fitted for volume reconstruction and for the computation of fire characteristics such as spread dynamics, local orientation, and heading direction.

Although it is already possible to extract some valuable fire development information by means of this stereo-vision-based technique, questions arise about its applicability in real-time scenarios without a priori knowledge of the fire. Furthermore, we believe that a grid-based approach is more appropriate than the ellipsoid modeling technique for fire development analysis, since interpretation and temporal analysis of the latter is not straightforward. Despite the limited results of the discussed video fire analysis approaches, the results from existing ordinary multiview object analysis approaches, such as the people and vehicle trackers in [11–13], are already very promising and their basics are also appropriate for video fire analysis. The majority of these works relies on homographic projection [14] of camera views, which also forms the basis of the FireCube framework described in [6].

The FireCube is a multiview localization framework that detects the 3D position and volume of the fire in an accurate manner. It is a prime example of how video-based detectors will be able to do more than just generate alarms, and should be seen as a first step in the direction of an application aiding firefighters in assessing the fire risk more efficiently.

Using this FireCube framework, information about the fire location and (growing) size can be generated very accurately and quickly. First, the framework detects the fire (ie, smoke or flames) in each single view. In order to do this, the framework uses some low-cost flame and smoke detectors (as discussed in Chapters 2 and 3). Secondly, the single-view detection results of the available cameras are projected by homography [14] onto horizontal and vertical planes which slice the scene, as shown in Fig. 4.3. For optimal

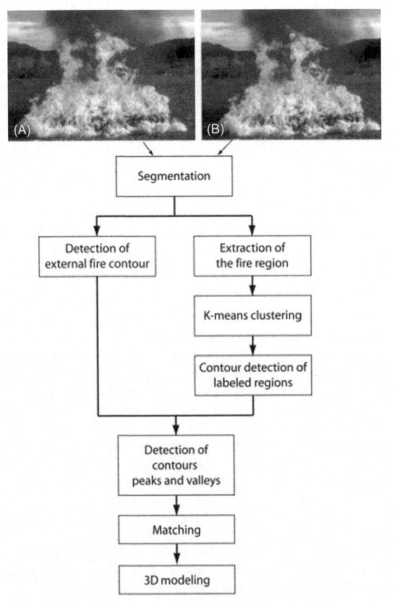

Figure 4.2 Video fire analysis system by Akhloufi and Rossi [7–9]: (A) input (stereo-vision) video sequences; (B) general scheme of 3D modeling framework;

(Continued)

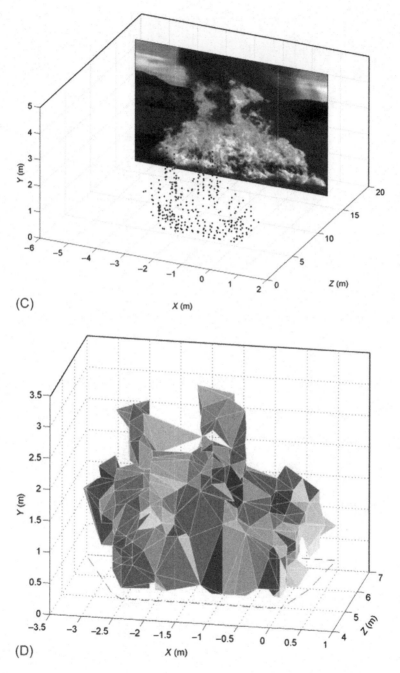

Figure 4.2, cont'd (C) 3D position of corresponding "feature points"; (D) 3D surface reconstruction of the fire.

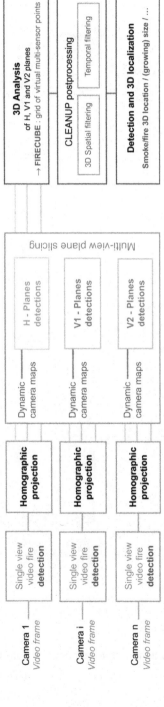

Figure 4.3 Global architecture of the FireCube multiview localization framework for 3D smoke and flame analysis.

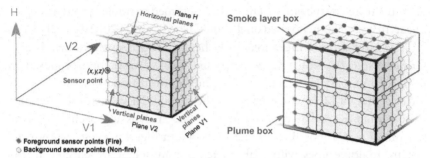

Figure 4.4 Generation of easily interpretable flame and smoke characteristics based on FireCube grid of foreground (FIRE) and background (NONFIRE) sensor points.

performance it is assumed that the camera views overlap such that each position is seen by at least two cameras. Overlapping multicamera views provide elements of redundancy (ie, each point is seen by multiple cameras) helping to minimize ambiguities like occlusions and improving the accuracy in the determination of the position and size of the flames and smoke. Next, the multiview plane slicing algorithm averages the multiview detection results in each of the horizontal and vertical planes. This step is a 3D extension of Arsic's multiple plane homography [15]. Then, a 3D grid of virtual multicamera sensors (ie, the FireCube) is created at the crossings of these planes.

At each sensor point of the 3D FireCube, the detection results of the horizontal and vertical planes that cross in that point are analyzed and only the points with stable detections are further considered as candidate fire or smoke. Finally, 3D spatial and temporal filters clean up the grid and remove the remaining noise. The filtered grid, shown in Fig. 4.4, can then be used to extract the smoke and fire location, information about the growing process and the direction of propagation.

Objective and subjective results of large-scale experiments, in which the flames and smoke development in a car park are analyzed [16], confirm these findings and indicate that the proposed multiview fire localization framework is able to accurately detect and localize the fire [17]. However, in its current form, the framework's computational complexity is not yet fully suitable for real-time processing and video-driven fire forecasting. For this reason, the next section discusses a multiview analysis set-up with lower processing cost, higher practical applicability, and only slightly less accuracy.

4.3 MULTIVIEW VIDEO FIRE ANALYSIS

Since most of the time we have multiple cameras monitoring the scene from different viewpoints, problems that arise in one camera can (most probably) be compensated by the others. This is also confirmed by smoke spreading experiments that we have performed on the multiview RABOT2012 dataset [18,19].

The estimation of the smoke layer height in each single camera is performed using the single view video fire analysis technique proposed in [20]. A commonly used technique for the determination of the smoke layer interface height [21], which relies on the second derivative of the temperature profile, is translated into a novel video analysis approach. A general scheme of the proposed algorithm is shown in Fig. 4.5. At start-up of the system, multiple lines with high energy are automatically selected in the video images. These lines show a strong similarity with thermocouples that are used for temperature profile analysis. The energy values $E_N^{line}[x, y]$ of these lines are calculated using the DWT-based energy calculation proposed by Calderara et al. [22]. At run-time, the energy profile EP_N^{line} is constructed by blockwise normalization of all the energy values in the energy line. In order to find the smoke layer depth, the gradient ∇EP^{line} of the energy profile is analyzed. The first point at which the gradient shows a high increase is labeled as the smoke layer depth. By subtracting this smoke layer depth from the height of the room, the smoke layer interface hint can be retrieved.

Based on the estimated h_{int} of all the camera views, we propose a multiview extension of the single-view algorithm based on the within- and between-variance of the multiview hint estimations. Figs. 4.6 and 4.7 show the estimated smoke height for TEST1 and TEST2 measured by two cameras with a different position and field of view. For each of these camera views, the chart contains the h_{int} values of three energy lines. Based on the differences between these h_{int} values, an indication on the accuracy of the measurements at each moment t in time can be given. For example, if the variance $\sigma_w(t)$ (Eq. [1]) on h_{int} is high within one of the camera views, it is less safe to trust the measurements of this view compared to a camera view in which the within-variance of hint is smaller. Furthermore, it is also important to check the between-variance $\sigma_b(t)$ (Eq. [2]) of the camera views, since this can give an indication regarding the certainty of the measurements. Fig. 4.8, for example,

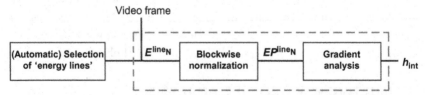

Figure 4.5 Generation of easily interpretable flame and smoke characteristics based on FireCube grid of foreground (FIRE) and background (NONFIRE) sensor points.

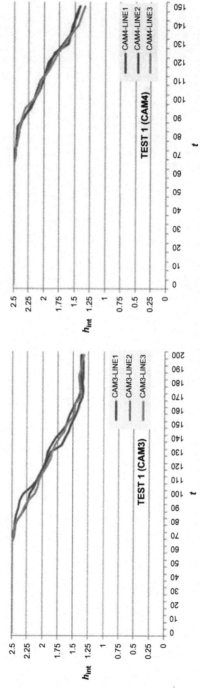

Figure 4.6 Smoke height in living—TEST1 (CAM3 vs. CAM4)—RABOT FIRE TESTS.

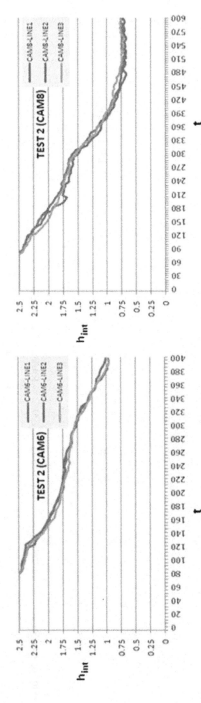

Figure 4.7 Smoke height in living—TEST2 (CAM6 vs. CAM8)—RABOT FIRE TESTS.

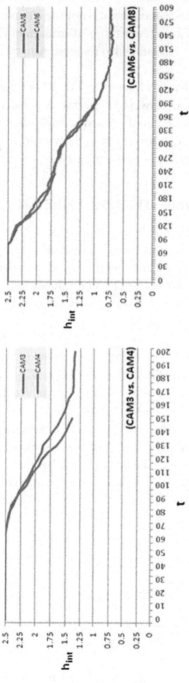

Figure 4.8 Smoke height in living—TEST1 vs. TEST2—RABOT FIRE TESTS.

shows that the average h_{int} values of CAM3 and CAM4 already separate at $t = 130$ s. This can be an indication that it is not safe anymore to trust the cameras. Contrary, for TEST2 we see that the estimations of CAM6 and CAM8 closely follow each other, indicating that their estimations can be trusted with high(er) probability.

The reason why we have a closer fit in TEST2 compared to TEST1 can be found in the fact that we lowered the cameras beneath the smoke layer. This has, of course, an impact on the practical applicability of the cameras in other applications (eg, video surveillance). However, to study/forecast the fire evolution in real-time, it has proven to be far more effective.

4.4 MULTIMODAL/MULTISENSOR FIRE ANALYSIS

As with any of the other fire detection technologies, video fire detection (VFD) is not immune to false alarms and missed detections. Insufficient lighting, steam, dust, and shadows, among others, lead to nuisance alarms or malfunctioning of the algorithms in VFD systems. In addition to these detection problems, misclassifications in VFD affect the retrieval of valuable video-based information about the fire scene (eg, smoke layer height and fire location) used for fire forecasting. In this section, we focus on both VFD limitations and investigate the gain achieved by combining volume sensors, like the Xtralis' OSID beam sensors, and SOTA VFD technologies [23]. By using sensors that don't depend on illumination and/or are immune to steam and dust, the VFD detection problems can be addressed directly. The novel multisensor approach leads to improved smoke alarm verification, smoke localization validation, and smoke layer depth measurement. Furthermore, due to its generic architecture, the proposed system can easily be adapted to other types of volume sensors.

A representation of the proposed multisensor combination and the algorithms interactions can be seen in Fig. 4.9. By integrating the output from

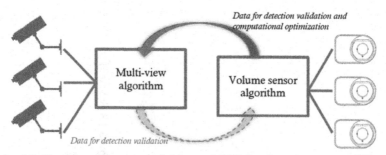

Figure 4.9 Algorithms interaction of video and OSID fire detection sensors [23].

OSID with the information from VFD, both detection systems share information (ie, giving feedback) to each other. For localizing the fire with the volume sensors, a 2D OSID MESH is introduced, whereas for the measurement of the smoke layer height, a linear array (of sensors) is implemented. Both set-ups are discussed in more detail in the next sections.

In order to test the new analysis techniques, we carried out real fire experiments in a car park at WarringtonFireGent. Both VFD detectors and volume sensor systems were used with different fires and set-ups. The first set of experiments focused on the 2D MESH smoke localization, which output (for example) can be used for adaptive mesh refinement in the existing 3D FireCube [6,17]. The second set of experiments was targeted to the OSID-based optimization of VFD smoke layer depth measurement. Results of both experiments are given later in this paper. First of all, we briefly discuss the OSID beam sensor (ie, the detector we have chosen to combine VFD with other volume sensors).

Several types of sensors could be considered for the combination with VFD. Point detectors, for instance could be useful in small, closed areas. However, for these types of areas there is not much benefit of VFD over other sensors. For the detection and forecast of fire in large, open spaces (such as car parks and atria), it is of a greater significance to combine VFD with volume sensors, like thermopile arrays, Light Detection and Ranging (LIDAR), and beam detectors. For testing our generic architecture, the latter volume sensor is chosen. However, similar results/benefits are expected with other combinations of volume sensors.

Traditional beam detectors are prone to generating false alarms due to object intrusion (eg, banners, balloons, insects, and birds) or dust within the path of the beam. These objects can cause the predefined light attenuation (or light scattering threshold) with a considerable probability, depending on the installation conditions, thus triggering nuisance alarms. OSID enhances the concept of the traditional beam detector and uses wide-angled beams containing sequences of ultraviolet (UV) and IR light pulses sent from an emitter with a unique coding, which are captured by an imager that compares the two types of light. A simplified representation of the operation of a single-emitter implementation of OSID is shown in Fig. 4.10. For OSID it is possible to discriminate between false positives and real smoke alarms, as the dust or intruding objects have bigger particles affecting both, the larger wavelength IR light and the shorter wavelength UV light, while the smaller particles of real smoke affect the UV light predominantly [24]. Its performance against nuisance alarms makes OSID a good type of detector to

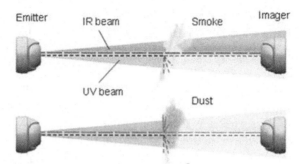

Figure 4.10 Linear OSID operation—simplified. *(Taken from R. Knox, Open-Area Smoke Imaging Detection (OSID). Suppression, Detection and Signaling Research and Applications—a Technical Working Conference (SUPDET), 2010, pp. 1–11).*

combine with VFD in order to overcome the false positives experienced by this technology, especially under difficult lighting conditions, or in the presence of shadows, smoke, or dust. Also, the possibility of covering wide areas (or volumes) with multiple emitters associated to a single imager makes OSID a suitable technology for the intended large, open spaces for the VFD system.

OSID detectors can be installed in several configurations, covering lines, areas, and even volumes. Depending on the configuration of these detectors, the algorithm proposed would be able to validate a smoke alarm, validate the location of the smoke, and/or supply information for the fire forecast (eg, the depth of the smoke layer). The two configurations that we propose are the OSID 2D MESH (for localization) and OSID ARRAY (for smoke layer depth analysis).

4.4.1 OSID 2D MESH

OSID detectors basically wait for any kind of medium interfering with the signal between the emitter and the imager and then by comparing between the UV and IR signal attenuation, decide if it is real smoke or something else. When the OSID imager detects smoke from any of the emitters associated to it, it raises an alarm and indicates from which emitter the detection was made. These alarm data are additionally used to detect the presence of smoke and locate it within the covered area.

The 2D OSID MESH, shown in Fig. 4.11A, makes use of dual OSID measurements by taking the crossing points between two sets of emitters associated to two different imagers. In the scheme, the symbols A_I and B_I correspond to the two imagers (ie, imager A and imager B) while the symbols A_n

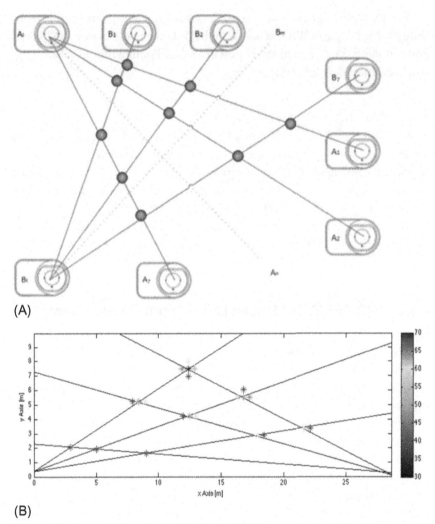

(A)

(B)

Figure 4.11 General example of (A) OSID 2D MESH in a rectangular-shaped room and (B) 2D MESH detections with time.

and B_m correspond to the emitter number n or m associated to the corresponding imager. Each imager can have up to 7 emitters associated. Then, given that all of the beams from one of the set of emitters cross the ones from the other (depending on the location of the detectors, some beams would not cross all of the other imager's associated beams) the amount of crossing points, C_P, is the product $C_P = N \times M$, where N is the amount of emitters associated to imager A and M is the amount of emitters associated to B.

For each point in 2D space (with coordinates x and y), its smoke probability value (P_{smoke}-OSID) is based on the distance to the closest 2D MESH point in alarm, r_{alarm}, and to the closest 2D MESH point without alarm, r_{clear}, and is calculated as follows:

$$P_{smoke\text{-}OSID} = \frac{r_{clear}}{r_{alarm} + r_{clear}}$$

The inclusion of P_{smoke}-OSID in a VFA framework, like in [25], can either lower down the average to correct a nuisance point or increase the average to correct a false negative. The information from the OSID detectors is used for confirming any initial detection alarm from the VFD. Furthermore, by implementing the 2D MESH, the initial location of the fire can be determined and the spread of the smoke at ceiling level (at an initial state) can be traced (Fig. 4.11B), thus providing useful information for multiview/multimodal fire analysis.

4.4.2 OSID ARRAY for Smoke Layer Depth Measurement

Unlike the 2D MESH set-up for the smoke detection and localization in which two different sets of OSID detectors were used in a horizontal, "planar," configuration, for the measurement of the smoke layer depth only one set of detectors is used. The emitters are placed vertically in a linear configuration forming an array of OSID emitters (ie, the OSID ARRAY). All of the emitters are associated to one same imager as shown in Fig. 4.12A and the first of the C_k (the emitters in the array) is the top one. The reference system for the location of the OSID detectors is based on the ceiling and the symbol z_k represents the distance between the ceiling and the kth emitter. The imager, C_I, should be located as low as or lower than the last of the emitters in the array (ie, the bottom one) so that the interruption by smoke of the signals between the imager and the emitter happens at the height of each emitter. The measurement of the smoke layer depth is done, thus, based on the location (height) of the emitters that go in alarm: the lowest of the emitters in the alarm determines the measured depth. Consequently, the growth of the smoke layer is not recorded continuously but rather discretely, at the measuring heights that correspond to the emitters. The values corresponding of the times in between should be estimated. As a first approach, a linear interpolation between each pair of values is proposed, as shown in Fig. 4.12B. More complex calculated values could be obtained by taking into account the rate of growth of the smoke layer according to previous points.

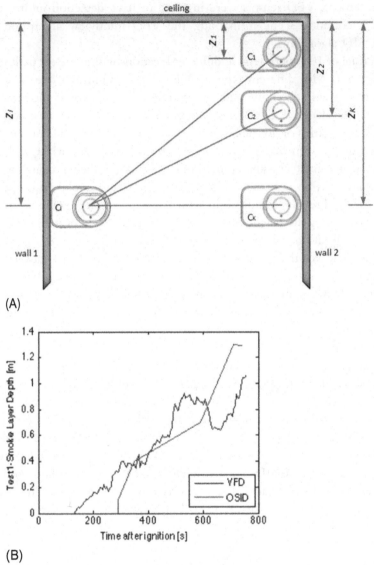

(A)

(B)

Figure 4.12 General example of (A) OSID ARRAY configuration and (B) comparison of 2D ARRAY and VFD detections with time.

4.4.3 OSID-VFD Experiments

The OSID 2D MESH and OSID ARRAY set-ups were tested in the construction were the Fire Safety and Explosion Safety in Car Parks [16] project took place. Two sets of experiments were performed: one for smoke detection and localization and another for the smoke layer depth measurement. VFD sensors were installed to have detection information from a common scene from both, the VFD multiview algorithm and the OSID algorithms.

A total of 10 experiments at different locations within the car park were carried out, with different types of fuels, (eg, fast burning ones like dry Christmas trees and straw, and smoldering ones like wood). For the 2D MESH, we analyzed the different moments in time in which new crossing points raise alarms or go back to normal status. From Fig. 4.11B, for example, it can be seen how the smoke is spread in the car park from being detected at a single crossing point until it covers all of the 9 crossing points. This way, it is possible to know the behavior of the smoke (at the initial stage of the fire). In combination with the VFD results, which were also collected during these experiments, further improvement of the FireCube's smoke localization results [6,17] is possible. The inclusion of P_{smoke}-OSID can either lower the average to correct a nuisance point or increase the average to correct a false negative. Furthermore, the 2D MESH detection results can also be used to determine in which areas of the FireCube it is important to have a higher accuracy. In this way, an adaptive, more targeted version of the FireCube can be created (ie, a possible direction for future work).

The second set of experiments performed in the car park was for the smoke layer depth measurement (Fig. 4.13). An OSID ARRAY of 5 emitters (shown in red (dark gray in print version)) was associated to 1 imager and 2 VFD cameras were used in addition to record the video needed to run the visual VFD approach [7]. A comparison of the 2D ARRAY and VFD smoke layer depth detections is shown in Fig. 4.13B. As can be seen, the continuous VFD and discrete OSID-based detection results have a rather good fit, and misdetections in each of the sensors can be corrected by the other one and vice versa. Similar OSID-VFD fits were also found for the other experiments.

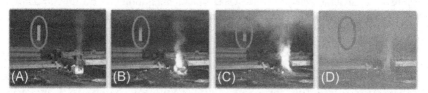

Figure 4.13 OSID-VFD smoke layer depth measurement experiments—Frames from Camera 1 during Test 1 after ignition at (A) 180 s, (B) 347 s, (C) 517 s, and (D) 880 s.

4.5 CONCLUSIONS

To avoid fire disasters, minimize damage, and save lives, early fire localization and detection of fire propagation are essential. Until now, however, no system existed capable of accurately detecting this valuable fire characteristics in real-time. In this chapter, we have introduced several multimodal/multisensor analysis techniques for the extraction and analysis of valuable fire character-istics, such as fire location, size, and growth.

It is important to remark that the VFA techniques proposed in this chapter are generally applicable (ie, they can easily be adapted when the environment changes or when they are applied in a slightly different scene). The experiments showed that the performance of the algorithms do not rely heavily on the type of building structure. Finally, it is also important to note that we impose the restrictions that the scene is intended to record using static cameras, that the cameras in a multiview setup overlap, and that the lines of sight of the cameras in a multimodal setup are close to each other.

Two different multisensor systems based on volume sensors (OSID) and cameras were introduced in this chapter, (ie, the 2D MESH and 2D ARRAY). Also, two new algorithms in charge of the processing of the information gathered by the OSID-based systems were presented. The novel OSID-based approaches lead to improved smoke alarm verification, smoke localization validation, and smoke layer depth measurement. Fur-thermore, due to its generic architecture, the proposed system can easily be adapted to other types of volume sensors and combined with VFD (or other sensors) in a multimodal setup.

REFERENCES

[1] R. Yasmin, Detection of smoke propagation direction using color video sequences, Int. J. Soft Comput. 4 (1) (2009) 45–48.
[2] J.R. Martinez-de Dios, J.C. Andre, J.C. Goncalves, B.C. Arrue, A. Ollero, D.X. Viegas, Laboratory fire spread analysis using visual and infrared cameras, Int. J. Wildland Fire 15 (2) (2006) 175–186.
[3] D.X. Viegas, M.G. Cruz, L.M. Ribeiro, A.J. Silva, A. Ollero, B. Arrue, R. Dios, F. Gmez-Rodrguez, L. Merino, A.I. Miranda, P. Santos, Gestosa fire spread experi-ments, in: Proceedings of IV International Conference on Forest Fire Research 2002, Wildland and Fire Safety Summit, 2002, pp. 1–13.
[4] J.R. Martinez-de Dios, B.C. Arrue, A. Ollero, L. Merino, F. Gomez-Rodriguez, Computer vision techniques for forest fire perception, Image Vis. Comput. 26 (4) (2008) 550–562.
[5] E. Pastor, A. Agueda, J. Andrade-Cetto, M. Munoz, Y. Perez, E. Planas, Computing the rate of spread of linear flame fronts by thermal image processing, Fire Saf. J. 41 (8) (2006) 569–579.

[6]   S. Verstockt, S. Van Hoecke, N. Tilley, B. Merci, B. Sette, P. Lambert, C. Hollemeersch, R. Van de Walle, FireCube: a multiview localization framework for 3D fire analysis, Fire Saf. J. 46 (5) (2011) 262–275.

[7]   L. Rossi, M. Akhloufi, Y. Tison, On the use of stereo vision to develop a novel instrumentation system to extract geometric fire fronts characteristics, Fire Saf. J. 46 (1-2) (2011) 9–20.

[8]   M. Akhloufi, L. Rossi, Three-dimensional tracking for efficient fire fighting in complex situations, in: Proceedings of the SPIE Visual Information Processing XVIII, Volume 7341, 2009, pp. 1–12.

[9]   L. Rossi, T. Molinier, M. Akhloufi, Y. Tison, A. Pieri, A 3D vision system for the measurement of the rate of spread and the height of fire fronts, Meas. Sci. Technol. 21 (10) (2010) 1–12.

[10] C. Schmid, R. Mohr, C. Bauckhage, Comparing and evaluating interest points, in: Proceedings of the 6th International Conference on Computer Vision, 1998, pp. 230–235.

[11] S.M. Khan, M. Shah, A multiview approach to tracking people in crowded scenes using a planar homography constraint, in: Proceedings of 9th European Conference on Computer Vision, 2006, pp. 133–146.

[12] S. Park, M. Trivedi, Homography-based analysis of people and vehicle activities in crowded scenes, in: Proceedings of the IEEE Workshop on Applications of Computer Vision, 2007.

[13] S. Verstockt, S. De Bruyne, C. Poppe, P. Lambert, R. Van de Walle, Multiview object localization in H.264/AVC compressed domain, in: Proceedings of the 6th IEEE International Conference on Advanced Video and Signal Based Surveillance, 2009, pp. 370–374.

[14] R. Hartley, A. Zisserman, Estimation—2D projective transformations, in: Multiple View Geometry in Computer Vision, second ed., Cambridge University Press, Cambridge, UK, 2004.

[15] D. Arsic, E. Hristov, N. Lehment, B. Hornler, B. Schuller, G. Rigoll, Applying multi layer homography for multi camera person tracking, in: Proceedings of the 2nd ACM/IEEE International Conference on Distributed Smart Cameras, 2008, pp. 1–9.

[16] B. Merci, Special issue fire safety journal on car park fire safety, Fire Saf. J. 57 (2013) 1–106.

[17] S. Verstockt, Multimodal Video Analysis for Early Fire Detection, PhD thesis, Ghent University, Belgium, 2011. 14.12.2011.

[18] S. Verstockt, T. Beji, B. Merci, R. Van de Walle, RABOT2012—presentation of a multiview video dataset of the full-scale ('Rabot') fire tests, in: 7th International Seminar on Fire and Explosion Hazards, 2013.

[19] RABOT2012 website, http://multimedialab.elis.ugent.be/rabot2012/.

[20] T. Beji, S. Verstockt, R. Van de Walle, B. Merci, On the use of real-time video to forecast fire growth in enclosures, Fire. Technol 50 (4) (2014) 1021–1040.

[21] N. Tilley, P. Rauwoens, B. Merci, Verification of the accuracy of CFD simulations in small-scale tunnel and atrium fire configurations, Fire Saf. J. 46 (2011) 186–193.

[22] S. Calderara, P. Piccinini, V. Cucchiara, Smoke detection in video surveillance: a MoG model in the wavelet domain, in: Proceedings of 6th International Conference in Computer Vision Systems (ICVS), 2008, pp. 119–128.

[23] L. Gonzales, Combining volume sensors with multimodal video analysis for fire detection and forecasting, Master thesis in the Erasmus Mundus Study Program—International Master of Science in Fire Safety Engineering, 30.06.2013, Ghent.

[24] R. Knox, Open-area smoke imaging detection (OSID), in: Suppression, Detection and Signaling Research and Applications—A Technical Working Conference (SUPDET), 2010, pp. 1–11.

[25] S. Verstockt, T. Beji, P. De Potter, S. Van Hoecke, B. Sette, B. Merci, R. Van de Walle, Video driven fire spread forecasting (f)using multimodal LWIR and visual flame and smoke data, Pattern Recogn. Lett. 34 (1) (2013) 62–69.

CHAPTER 5

Conclusions

An overview of emerging signal, image, and video processing methods and techniques for fire detection is presented in this book. Cameras and infrared sensors are capable of monitoring large volumes. Fire detection methods for visible and infrared range cameras are described and compared to each other in terms of detection performance. Wildfire detection methods using stationary cameras and mobile platforms are also investigated.

A nonconventional, PIR-based flame detection system and comparative results with other sensing modalities are presented, as well. It is experimentally observed that video-based systems detect fire and smoke before PIR-based systems. However the false-alarm rate of PIR sensors are much lower than visible range cameras. Both surveillance cameras and PIR-based systems, being a cost-effective choice can complement readily available smoke detectors installed in buildings, and may be employed for uncontrolled flame detection purposes.

Apart from fire detection systems, methods and techniques for fire localization and propagation estimation are discussed. A real-time system capable of localizing fire and analyzing fire characteristics such as size and growth is presented.

Utilization of nonconventional, multi-modal, multi-sensor systems for fire detection and modeling fire behavior based on signal, image, and video processing techniques help pave the way for developing better, more efficient, and effective firefighting and mitigation strategies. Authors hope that this book focusing on recent volume sensing methods provides an introduction to this exciting field.

Methods and Techniques for Fire Detection
http://dx.doi.org/10.1016/B978-0-12-802399-0.00005-3

INDEX

Printed in the United States
By Bookmasters